HANDMADE HELPS FOR DISABLED LIVING

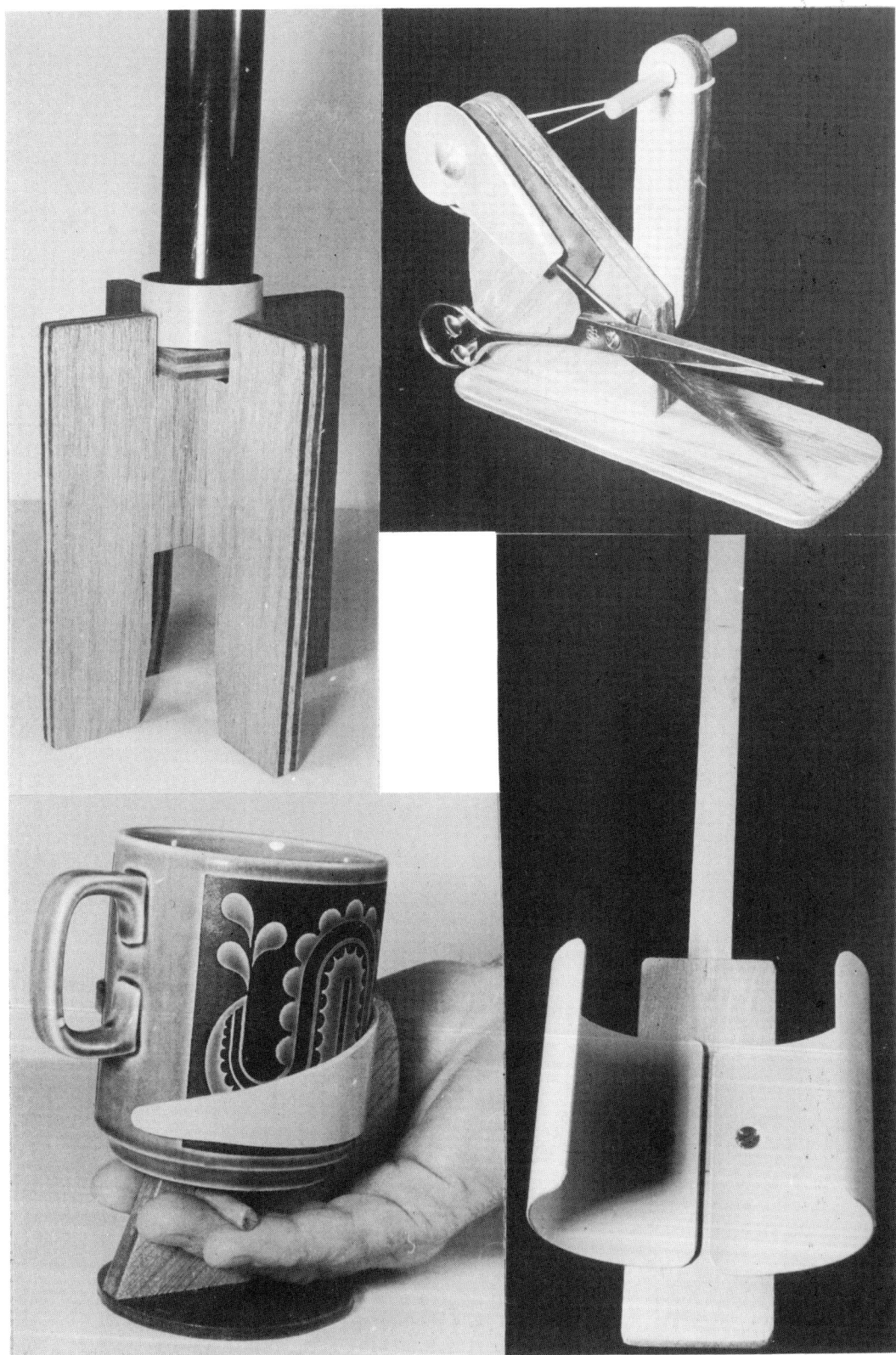

HANDMADE HELPS FOR DISABLED LIVING

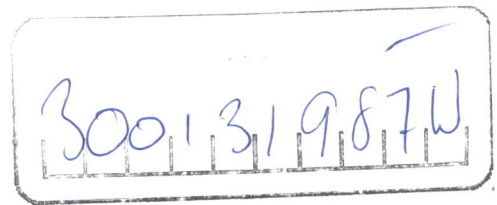

Stuart E. Grainger

B. T. Batsford London

First published as *Making Aids for Disabled Living* 1981
© Stuart E. Grainger 1981
This Edition First Published 1990
© Stuart E. Grainger 1990

ISBN 7134 3935 1

Printed in Great Britain by
Courier International Ltd
Tiptree, Essex
for the publishers
B.T. Batsford Ltd,
4 Fitzhardinge Street,
London W1H 0AH

Contents

Foreword

However well we look after ourselves, very few of us will be fortunate enough to leave this world without having encountered some kind of physical disability at some stage in our lives. It may be only the temporary annoyance of a broken bone, or a more prolonged trial by slipped disc, rheumatism or arthritis, but most people prefer to imagine that disability will never happen to them, vain though that hope may be. An unfortunate few have to live throughout their lives with permanent disabilities and their experience can be of great benefit to the rest of us when our turn comes to need help.

Social workers, occupational therapists and others, whose job it is to help and advise the disabled and handicapped, know well that the commercially produced aids, which they can offer to their clients, are not always well-suited to the needs of particular individuals, even if the money is available, and often it is not. Such aids are not cheap to buy, and yet many perhaps more satisfactory aids are simple enough to be made with hand tools on a kitchen table. Money is frequently spent on a costly device that can do no more than partially satisfy a need, when that need could be met more efficiently by an item specially produced in the well-equipped workshop of a local school. It would be of great social and educational benefit to all concerned if a greater effort was made to establish and encourage regular contact between centres for the handicapped and schools, adult education centres and colleges of further education. Often these establishments are close neighbours but never realise how much good they can do for each other. The benefits resulting from such contact are by no means in one direction only. Perhaps the greatest challenge faced by any teacher is the need to motivate pupils. Where design and technical skills are to be learned, what better motivation can there be than the alleviation of distress and suffering in the less fortunate?

What follows is a collection of designs for aids, which have been made over a period of several years in response to requests from various directions. Some of them appeared in a previous book, *Making Aids for Disabled Living*, which stimulated requests for more designs. Nearly all of the devices described here were originally designed and made for a particular person with a particular disability, but subsequently they have proved useful to many people with all kinds of disability and some with no disability at all. Several items appearing in this book are by no means exclusively for the use of handicapped people.

You do not need to be a medical expert or an engineer to produce what is wanted to solve the vast majority of problems faced by the disabled. You do need to be willing to listen and to use an unlimited amount of imagination. Often a problem is not quite what it seems to be at first inspection, nor is your first solution likely to be the perfect answer you thought it was. Be prepared to persevere, with repeated modifications to suit that particular case. Try to approach every problem with an open mind, without preconditions of any kind, other than the inevitable financial ones. Often an ideal aid can be produced by using a simple everyday object in a novel or unconventional way.

I once spent many hours of thought and experiment in an attempt to produce something which would enable a lady, whose hands were crippled by arthritis, to wring out a dishcloth, so she could carry out the normal task of wiping clean the working top in her kitchen. Several complicated and less than satisfactory devices were produced and rejected in turn, before the simplest of solutions suggested itself, whilst I watched her make some pastry. A rolling pin applied, not to pastry, but to a wet dishcloth on the draining board, produces the same effect as that of an old-fashioned mangle. We gave her a short length of plastic drainpipe, with which to roll out her dishcloth, and she was happier with that than with any of the far more expensive and carefully engineered prototypes offered previously. The moral of that story, of course, is 'Keep It Simple'. The more complicated and sophisticated a device is, the less it is likely to be used.

Some of these designs are more than ten years old and it may well be possible to improve them with the use of more up-to-date materials and tools. The 'Do It Yourself' market has flourished in recent times, and many new products and materials have appeared, which expand the opportunities and scope of the amateur inventor. There are many more plastic extrusions available now, not only in the form of water pipes of both round and square section, but angle bar, channel and other complex sections of various sizes sold for a variety of purposes, notably secondary double glazing with transparent plastic sheet. The arrival in recent years of hot-glue guns and hot-air guns has made it possible for the handyman to work thermoplastic extrusions and sheet in ways that have yet to be fully explored. This is a valuable new asset in the making of aids for the disabled, because it is so important that such devices are washable and plastic is eminently suitable for this reason alone.

It is freely acknowledged that the designs in this book are not necessarily the best answers to the problems they purport to solve, but at least they do offer an attempt at a solution. There are plenty more such problems waiting to be solved and I hope that my readers will provide matching solutions of their own. There may be little money in it, but there is much satisfaction to be gained thereby!

Handmaking

In producing these designs for publication, the aim has been to give priority to clarity, often at the expense of strict engineering drawing rules. If no scale is stated, it may be assumed that the drawing is full size. It is accepted by the author that the average reader making an aid from one of these designs will prefer to take a tracing from the drawings in the book, rather than redraw them himself, even though the dimensions are stated.

A second aim has been to ensure that, using these instructions, the aids can be made from readily obtainable materials, using standard tools in the normal way, by anyone with an average layman's skill in handling such tools. The tool kit required is quite basic and would include the following items:

hand saw or tenon saw	chisel
coping saw	vice
junior hacksaw	carpenter's rule
screwdrivers	pencils
sharp knife	chinagraph pencil or fibretip pen
hand drill and bits	
hammer	pair of pliers
coarse and fine glass-paper	warding files
	'G' cramps
pair of scissors	snips

A few other items may be found useful; for instance a pop-riveting tool, power drill, jigsaw and hot-glue gun would speed up production, but are not essential.

Materials

Very few of the dimensions stated are critical (where they are, the fact is clearly noted) and other materials than those suggested would often do as well. When considering a design, therefore, bear in mind what materials you already have available in the form of leftovers and offcuts, and ask yourself whether these would serve the purpose, even if they are not precisely as specified. The experienced amateur maker of aids becomes an inveterate squirrel, hoarding all kinds of unlikely odds and ends, bits and pieces, in the sure knowledge that, sooner or later, they will come in handy.

A certain amount of scrounging is often preferable to straightforward purchase, because buying a two-metre length of plastic drainpipe when you only want 50 millimetres is to be avoided if possible. In such a case try calling at a local builder's yard and offer to buy offcuts of a suitable size. If you can honestly claim that it is wanted to make an aid for a handicapped person, the charge is unlikely to be exorbitant and it may well be waived. A plumber or joiner may be willing to save offcuts for you, which are of no use to him, but which may be just what is needed for a cup-holder or tap spanner. Rubber from old motor car or bicycle tyre inner tubes can be most useful in all sorts of ways, so try and make friends at a local garage or tyre depot.

It is impossible to state definite sources of supply for materials, particularly on an international basis, but there is nothing at all exotic specified in this book and most handymen have their own favourite sources for items such as plywood, plastic pipe or sheet, screws and bolts. Any good 'Do It Yourself' store should be able to supply what is suggested, but the reader is urged to remember that these are truly only suggestions and that alternatives abound.

Several devices described in this book require screws and bolts, for which sizes are specified; however, it is not always easy to find a specific size of screw or bolt in retail outlets, so again, do remember that you do not need to have precisely what the book suggests, as long as what you use does the job required of it. A small difference in diameter will usually be of no consequence, but length could be important, so make sure any error is on the long side. An overlong bolt or screw can be trimmed down with a hacksaw and file, but one that is too short can not be stretched. In one or two cases, brand names have been mentioned, such as Meccano bolts or Copydex glue, but it should not be supposed that other bolts or glues will not do as well. The names were used because that is what was used in the original device. The small Meccano bolts are about 4 mm ($\frac{5}{32}$ in.) diameter and about 7 mm ($\frac{9}{32}$ in.) long. The plastic bolts are about 9 mm ($\frac{3}{8}$ in.) diameter, available in various lengths. Where plastic bolts have been specified, it is mainly because they will not corrode, but other brass, plastic or plated bolts will resist corrosion equally well. Copydex is a glue that is particularly good for application on fabric, where it can replace sewing, but other glues having a latex base can be equally effective in this role. Glue technology is improving all the time, so additional and probably better possibilities are likely to become available. As a general rule, if a brand name mentioned here is not familiar to you, ignore it and concentrate upon the purpose for which it is intended.

Washable finish

It is inevitable that some compromises have to be made in designing an article to be produced in a home instead of a factory. One area of compromise has been in the vital need to provide a washable finish on wooden items, which in a commercial product would have been moulded in plastic. Many forms of plastic sheet are now available on the DIY market, and these can be used to provide a washable surface for some items, the **Folding Bed Table** for instance, but this is by no means a universal possibility, even if the rather high cost were acceptable. Fortunately modern paints and varnishes provide excellent, hard-wearing and washable surfaces, so, although a little more care and labour are needed, the finished product is not inferior – indeed it often has a better appearance and has the advantage that it can always be repainted and thus rejuvenated.

Metrication

Many of these designs were orginally prepared at a time when a transition from feet and inches to the metric system was at an early stage in the United Kingdom. Unfortunately it is still not complete, with the result that one may have to order a sheet of 12 millimetre plywood 8 feet by 4 feet! No doubt other countries are less confused, but, to try and maintain a sense of order in this book, where measurements have been stated, equivalents have been included, although these sometimes appear slightly strange. The actual hardware from which a prototype device was made may well have been a mixture of measurements in both inches and millimetres. Thus a plastic water pipe of a standard 4-inch diameter appears in the drawings as having an equivalent diameter of 101 mm – the nearest approximation. If you live in an area where a similar pipe is of a standard 10 cms diameter, you may safely ignore the missing millimetre.

Similarly the sizes of plywood and prepared hardwood have been stated in the drawings to the nearest actual size in millimetres. At the time of writing, one still can buy prepared hardwood lengths, for instance, nominally of $\frac{1}{2}$-inch-square section, which actually measures 12 mm square. The dimensions given in this book have been measured from real items and are stated in real, not nominal, terms. To avoid any confusion, therefore, take a rule with you when buying hardware or materials and measure items for yourself before you pay for them; it can save a great deal of aggravation.

Hot glue and hot air

A hot-glue gun is a most useful tool, capable not only of gluing and sealing, but can also be valuable in laying down successive thicknesses of plastic glue, which set to a semi-rigid consistency and therefore can be used to form a ridge or knob precisely where one may be needed. The possession of a hot-air gun, normally used for paint stripping, is a further asset in conjuction with a hot-glue gun, because, once the glue has set, it can be heated on the surface, using the hot-air gun, and can be manipulated and shaped with an appropriate tool, such as an artist's palette knife, frequently dipped in water to avoid sticking. The hot-air gun can be used repeatedly to keep the plastic glue at a malleable temperature until the required shape is achieved. Do not try shaping it with your fingers, or you may easily be burned. Remember, when using a hot-air gun for this purpose, that it can easily scorch wood and set inflammable materials alight, so take proper care how you use it. Do not direct the hot air at one place continuously, but play it repeatedly backwards and forwards across the surface being worked, so that the temperature is raised evenly.

This technique can also be used to good effect for enlarging small handles, knobs and caps, or changing a round, slippery shape into a square or hexagonal shape that is much easier to hold and manipulate.

Another very valuable use for a hot-air gun is the reshaping of plastic piping or plastic sheet. For this purpose it is again most important that the heat is applied evenly and without scorching the material. Usually the gun may be held several inches away from the material being worked. Much depends upon the job being attempted, but often it is necessary to use a rough former upon which plastic can be shaped as it heats and becomes malleable. In the case of sheet, this may be a length of metal bar or rod over which the plastic can be bent in a straight line. Similarly metal tubing of an appropriate diameter can be used as a former upon which heated plastic sheet can be gradually rolled into a cylindrical or curved shape. Plastic water pipe and guttering, made from PVC, ABS, polyethylene, polypropylene or other material suitable for extrusion, can be softened in the same way as flat plastic sheet, using a hot-air gun, and the walls worked in much the same way, but manipulating the entire section of a pipe or tube, so as to bend it and retain rigidity after cooling is a much more difficult proposition. Attempting to do so is not recommended as consistency of shape and strength is almost impossible to attain without much more sophisticated equipment than is considered here.

Simple enough to be overlooked

There are several beautifully simple aids which are immediately available in most homes, so simple that they are often overlooked. Such items as clothes pegs and Bulldog paper clips have numerous uses in addition to those for which they were designed, particularly in the field of handicrafts. Two large Bulldog clips can be bolted together, through the holes in the finger grips, so that they are fixed back to back and thus provide the means of clamping almost anything of moderate size to a table, desk, chair or clothing, for example. Clamp the lower clip to a heavy weight, such as a lump of lead or iron, and you have a stable miniature vice or stand, for holding anything from macrame cords to a fishing fly. Ordinary bottle corks, with a suitable hole drilled longitudinally through the centre, offer a simple means of improving the grip of a weak or crippled hand upon such tools as knitting needles and crochet hooks.

Other potentially simple solutions to problems may be found in such items as rubber bands, double-sided adhesive tape, magnetic self-adhesive tape available for secondary double-glazing, self-adhesive Velcro tape, small magnets and the host of little gadgets that are constantly appearing in shops, advertisements and catalogues.

Keep your imagination finely tuned to possibilities beyond those which the designer intended. The habit of automatically evaluating every available article, particularly those which cost nothing, such as disposable containers, caps, bottles, bungs, boxes, tubes, covers and cartons for alternative uses is a fascinating and precious acquisition. Those who take the trouble to train their eyes to see will find that our society throws away great riches every day.

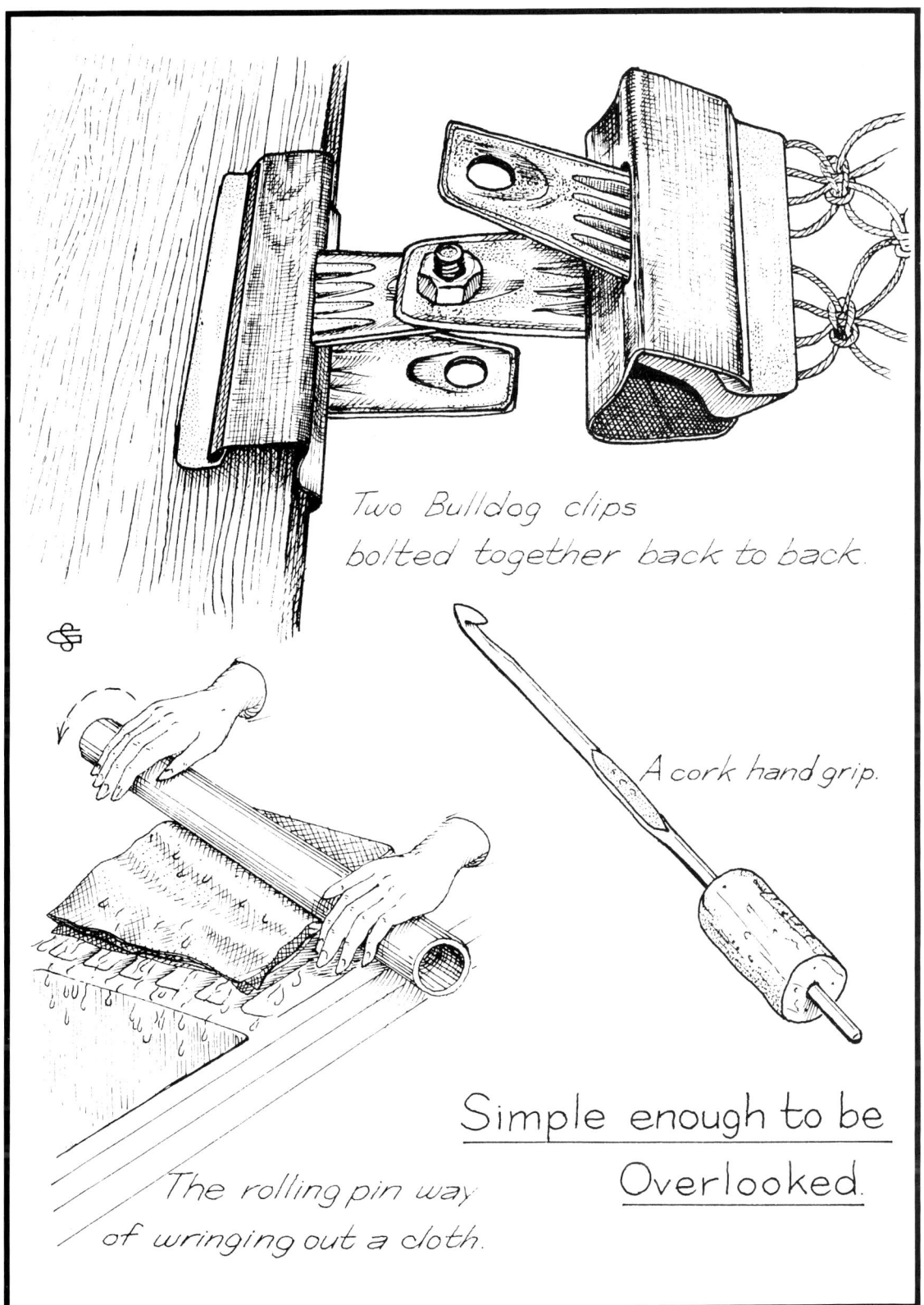

Two Bulldog clips
bolted together back to back.

A cork hand grip.

The rolling pin way
of wringing out a cloth.

Simple enough to be
Overlooked.

TAP SPANNERS

There are several ways of making tap spanners, and one of the simplest is merely to cut an appropriately shaped hole in a piece of plywood or metal provided with a suitable handle. The aforementioned method produces a spanner which cannot be left in place, however, for it will drop down onto the stem of the tap; it can also be difficult to position on some modern moulded plastic taps. The designs of tap spanners offered here are both very easy to make and one or other of them will fit all the taps that the author has encountered in recent years. It is necessary to provide two designs, one for taps with an even number of spokes, which is the large majority, and one for the minority having an uneven number of spokes.

Construction

Making these tap spanners is simplicity itself, consisting of just four steps:

1 Cut out the horizontal member from 12 mm ($\frac{15}{32}$ in.) plywood, using coping saw or jigsaw.
2 Drill the appropriately positioned holes for the pegs.
3 Cut the dowelling pegs 50 mm (2 in.) x 8 mm ($\frac{5}{16}$ in.) diameter.
4 Place a little wood glue in each hole and tap the pegs into place with a mallet.

The application of varnish or paint will help to protect the wood, but is not essential, particularly if marine quality plywood is used.

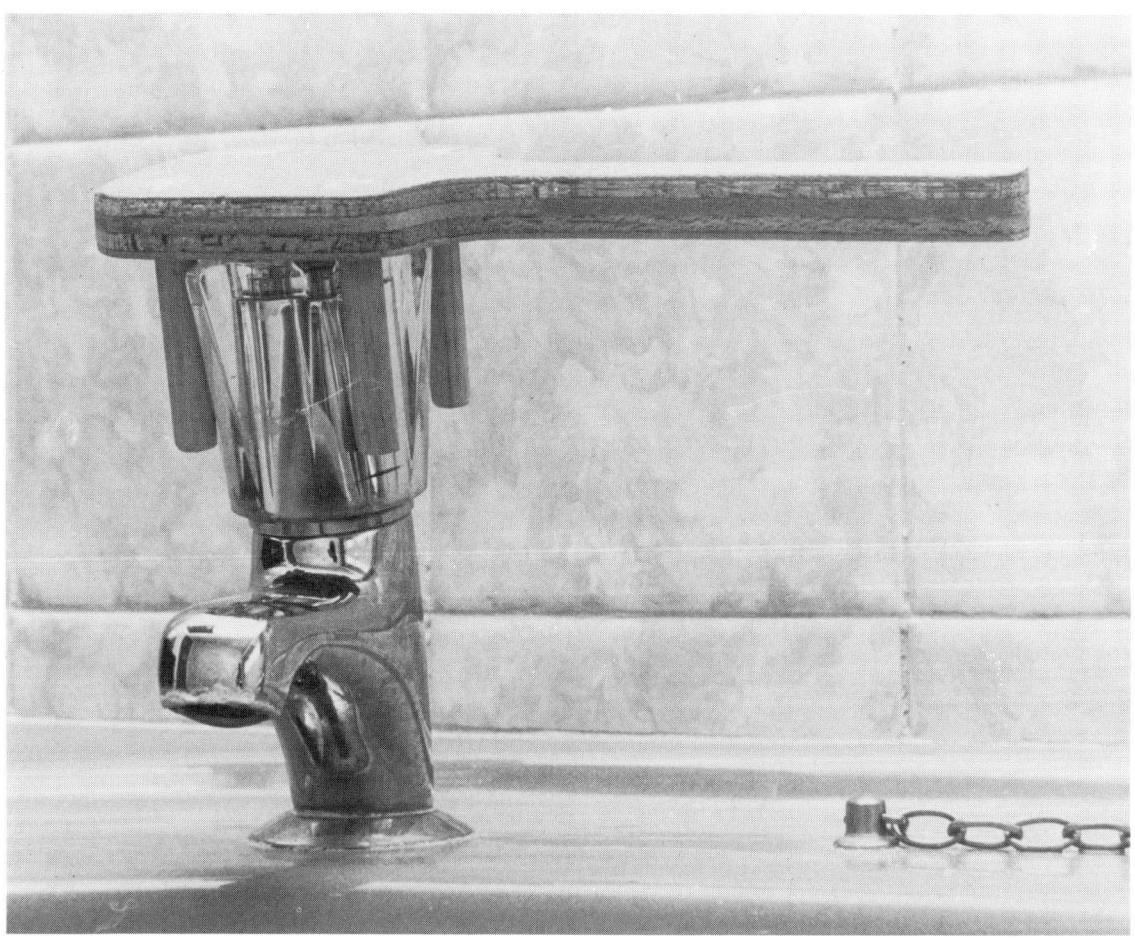

A Tap Spanner in position

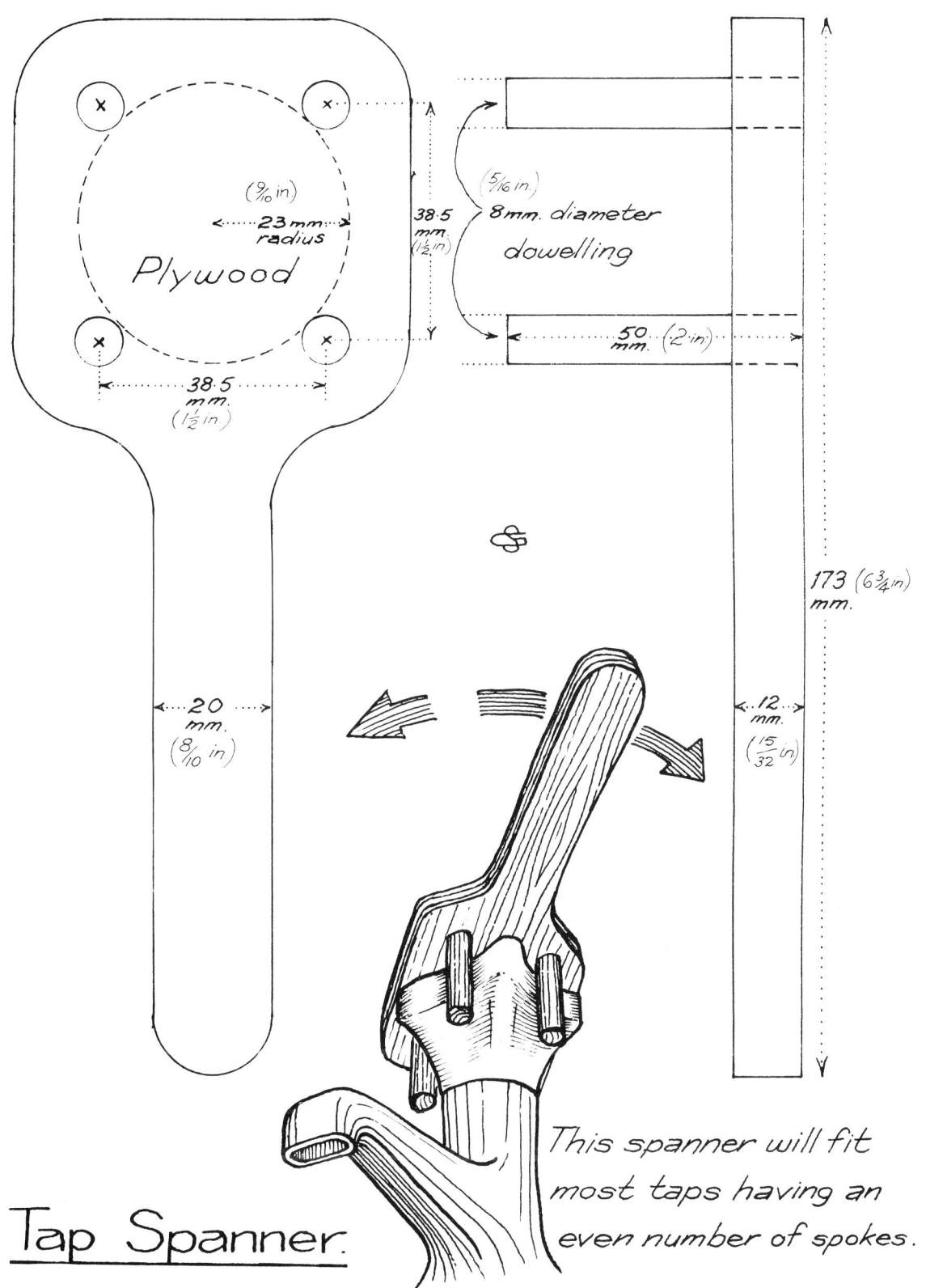

(9⁄10 in)

←·····23 mm.·····→
radius

Plywood

38.5
mm
(1½ in)

←········ 38.5 ········→
mm.
(1½ in)

(5⁄16 in.)

**8mm. diameter
dowelling**

←········ 50 (2 in) ········→
mm.

173 (6¾ in)
mm.

←··· 20 ···→
mm.
(8⁄10 in)

←··· 12 ···→
mm.
(15⁄32 in)

Tap Spanner.

*This spanner will fit
most taps having an
even number of spokes.*

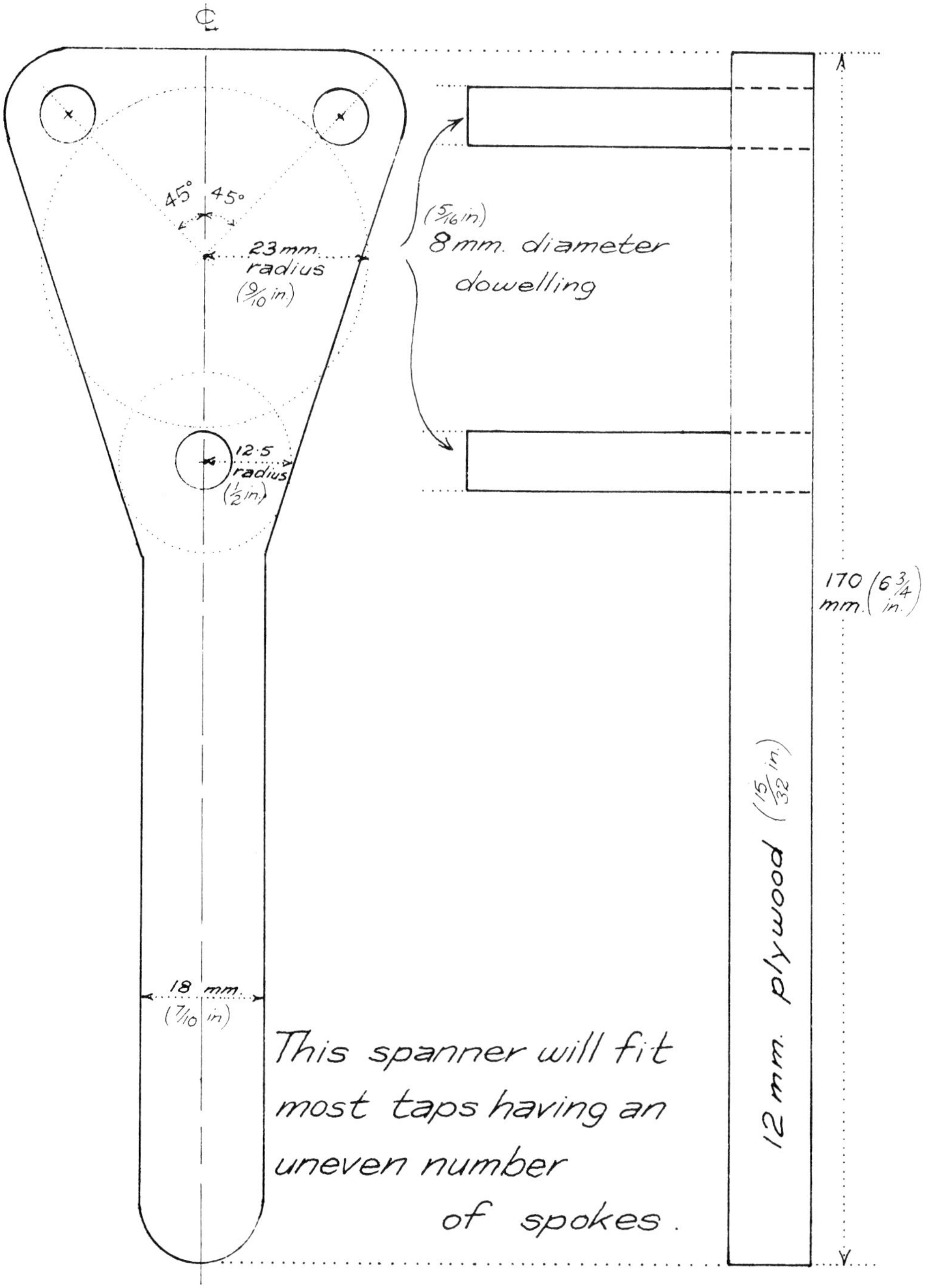

Ȼ

45° 45°

23 mm.
radius
(9/10 in.)

12.5
radius
(1/2 in.)

(5/16 in.)
8 mm. diameter
dowelling

170 (6 3/4
mm.   in.)

12 mm. plywood (15/32 in.)

18 mm.
(7/10 in.)

This spanner will fit
most taps having an
uneven number
                of spokes.

Tap Spanner II.

TOE TOUCHER

Those who find it difficult or impossible to reach their feet, and there are a great many of them, can face problems in trying to wash and to dry their toes, which may eventually cause complications. A very simple aid to overcoming these problems may be provided by taking a piece of 12 mm ($\frac{1}{2}$ in.) diameter hardwood dowelling 450 to 600 mm (18 to 24 in.) long and cutting a slot about 2 mm ($\frac{3}{32}$ in.) wide through the lower end of it, extending about 150 mm (6 in.) up the length. The split end is then rounded off and sanded perfectly smooth.

This makes a kind of extended dolly-peg. The corner or edge of a towel or wash cloth can be inserted into the slot, rolled up for a turn or two and may then be used as a finger extension to wash or dry around and between the toes.

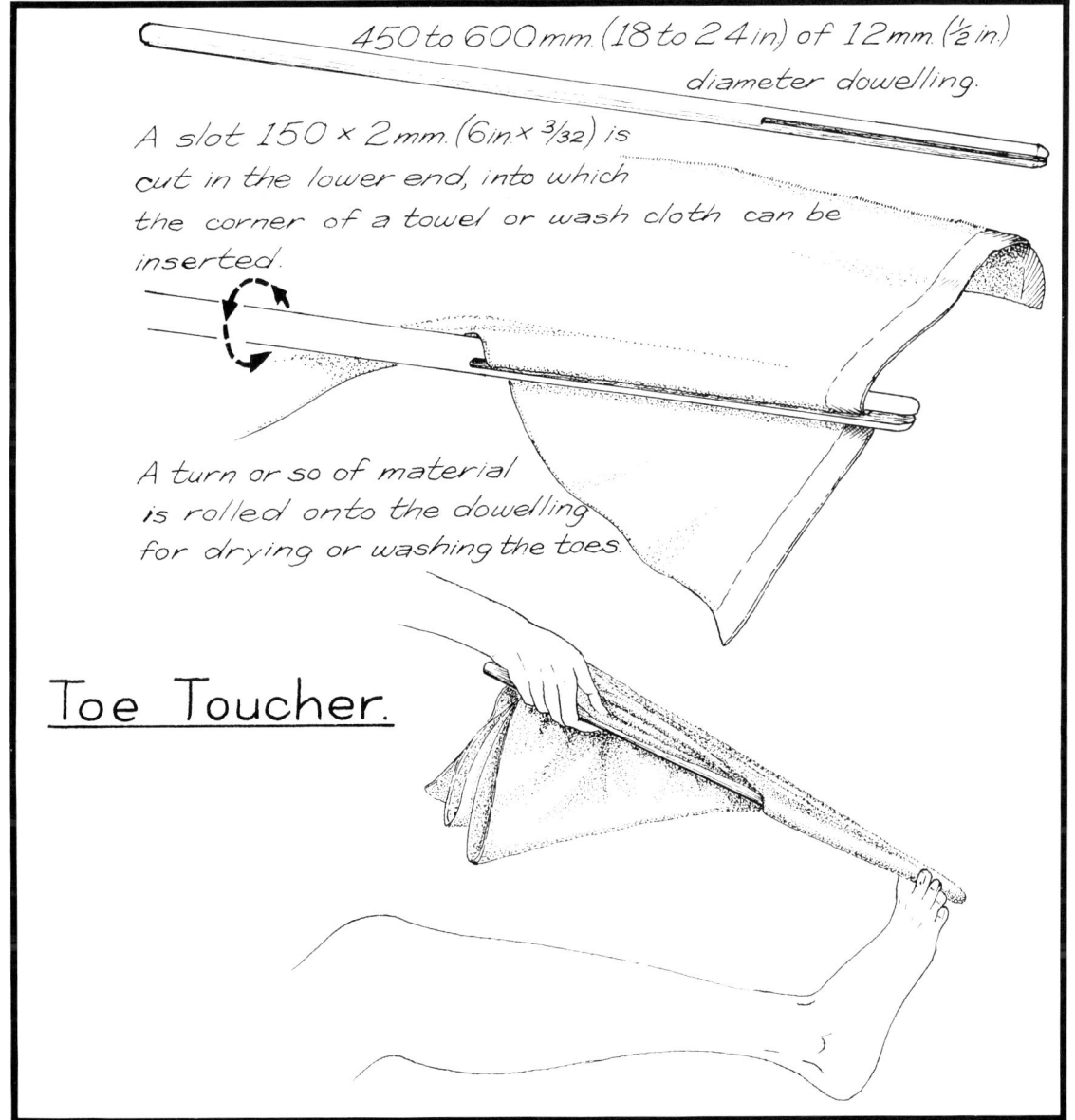

450 to 600mm. (18 to 24 in) of 12mm. (½ in.) diameter dowelling.

A slot 150 × 2mm. (6in.× 3/32) is cut in the lower end, into which the corner of a towel or wash cloth can be inserted.

A turn or so of material is rolled onto the dowelling for drying or washing the toes.

Toe Toucher.

15

SOAP AND SPONGE MITT

These can be worthwhile items in any household, because they provide a very practical way of using up the small leftover pieces of soap that are usually thrown away. For anyone with limited use of their hands, or with only one hand, the Mitt is a most valuable washing aid. A hand can be slipped into it very easily and the soap inside it is precisely where it is needed when it is needed and cannot slip away, as it so easily will from a wet hand.

The Mitt is simplicity itself to make and is very inexpensive. It is made from the readily available and inexpensive plastic foam sheet, usually between 6 and 8 mm ($\frac{1}{4}$ to $\frac{5}{16}$ in.) thick, which is sold for dressmaking and quilting. The foam is open cell in form, which means that the bubbles in it are interconnecting and therefore act like a natural sponge, allowing water to pass from cell to cell. Unlike a natural sponge, however, plastic foam does not become unpleasantly slimy when used with soap. Since air will pass through the foam as readily as water does, the Mitt can be squeezed out and left in the bathroom to dry with the soap still inside it.

The method of construction is shown clearly in the drawings. It is merely a matter of folding a strip of the foam about 500 mm (20 in.) long by about 125 mm (5 in.) wide into three layers and sewing it together along the edges with button thread. It can even be glued if sewing is beyond you.

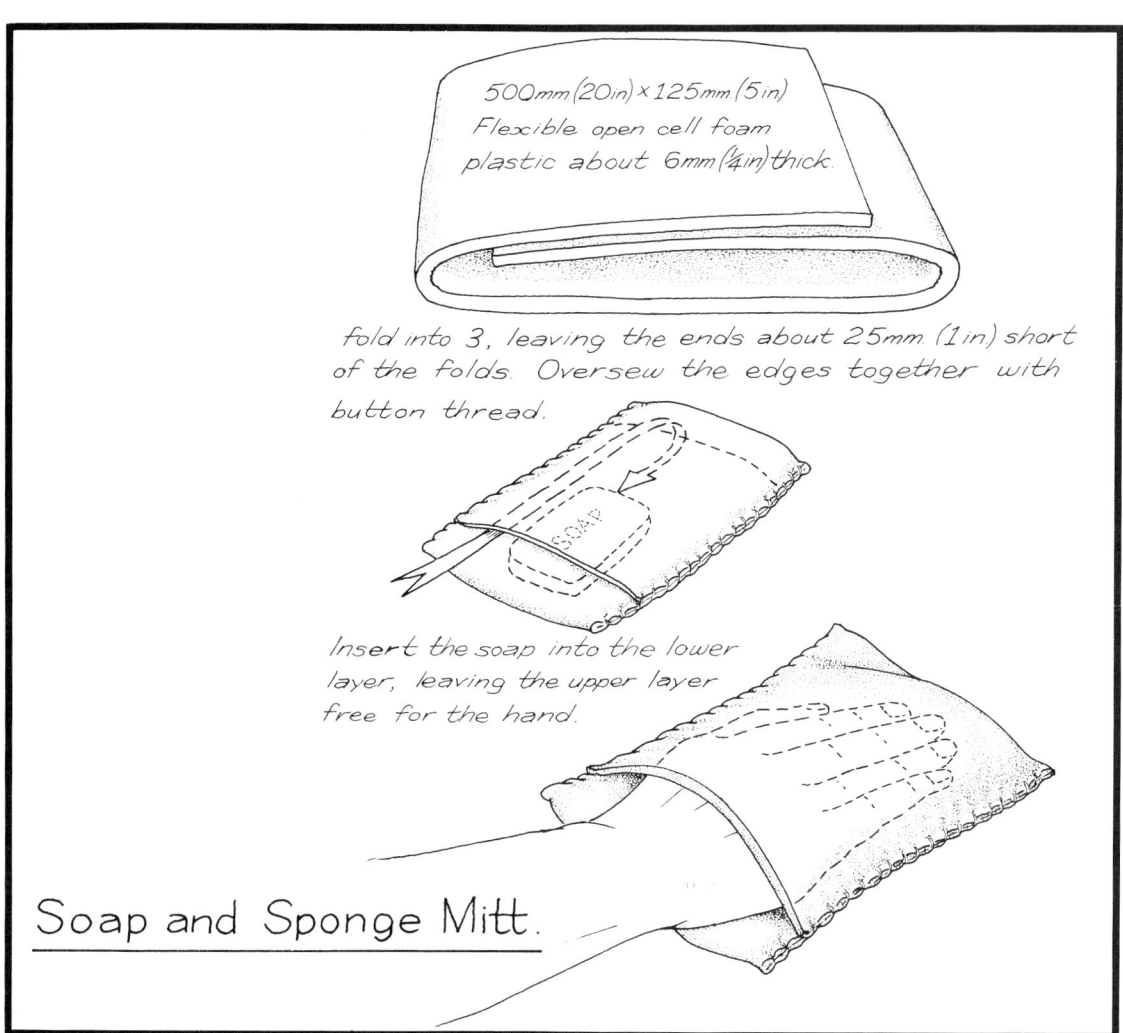

500mm (20in) x 125mm (5in)
Flexible open cell foam
plastic about 6mm (¼in) thick.

fold into 3, leaving the ends about 25mm. (1 in) short of the folds. Oversew the edges together with button thread.

Insert the soap into the lower layer, leaving the upper layer free for the hand.

Soap and Sponge Mitt.

REVERSIBLE DUAL HEIGHT RAISING BLOCKS

These blocks are intended for placing beneath the legs of a bed or other furniture which requires raising, so four such blocks are normally needed. Depending on which way up the blocks are placed, as illustrated in the diagrams they will lift the bed by either 110 mm ($4\frac{5}{16}$ in.) or 160 mm ($6\frac{5}{16}$ in.). Each block is formed by a pair of interlocking rectangular uprights, which are identical except for the vertical slots providing the means of interlocking them at right angles. A square block, conveniently available from the cut-away area of one of the uprights, bears the direct thrust from the furniture leg and transfers it evenly to the uprights. A short (about 50 mm, 2 in) length of PVC drainpipe of about 51 mm (2 in.) outside diameter rests on top of the bearing block to provide a locating collar, which prevents any possibility of the furniture leg slipping off the uprights.

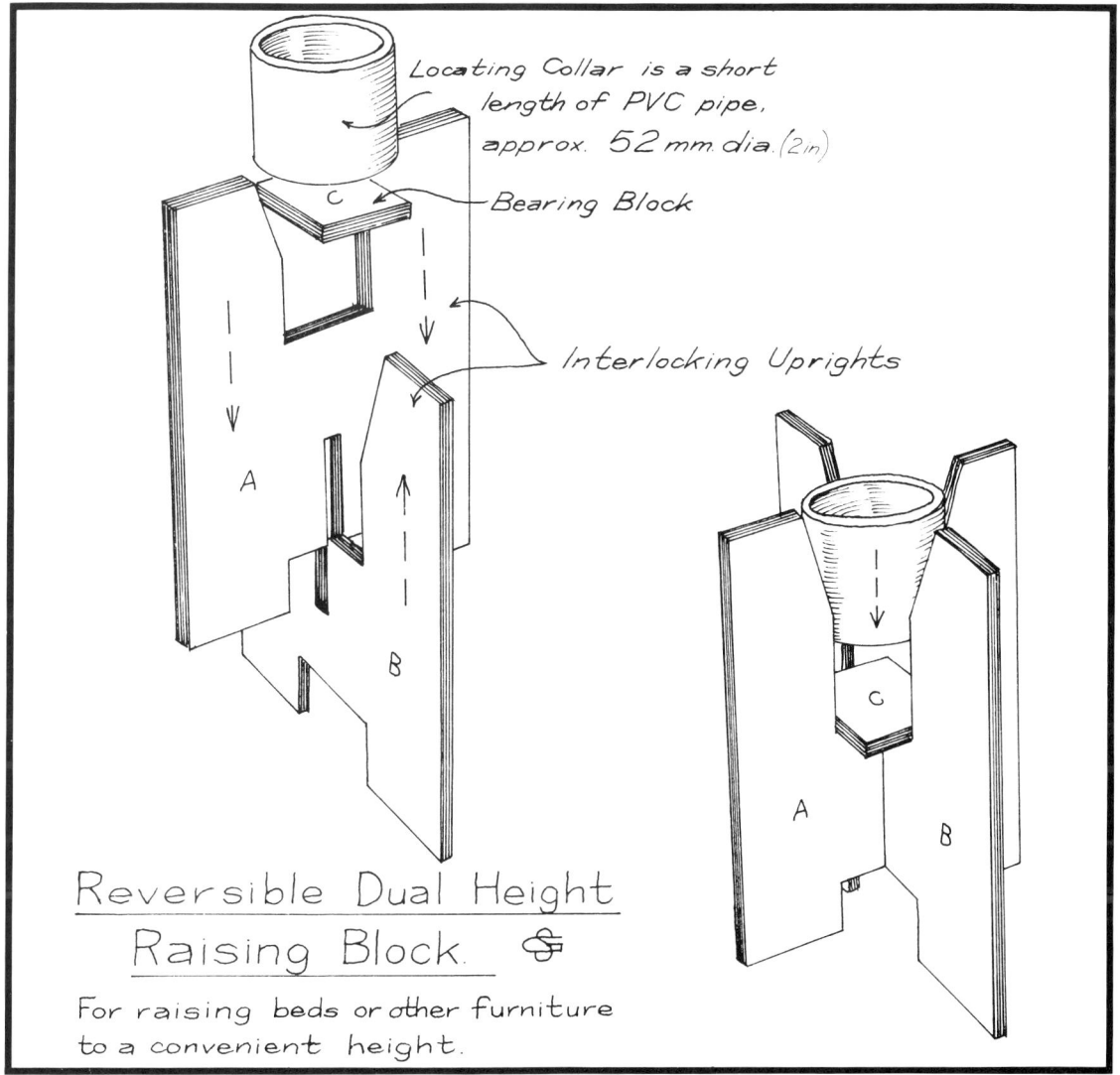

Locating Collar is a short length of PVC pipe, approx. 52 mm. dia. (2 in)

Bearing Block

Interlocking Uprights

Reversible Dual Height Raising Block.

For raising beds or other furniture to a convenient height.

It is not really necessary to paint or varnish the completed blocks, but it may be sensible to do so if they are likely to require washing regularly. If they are painted or varnished, ensure that the interlocking vertical slots are kept sufficiently free to slide and interlock.

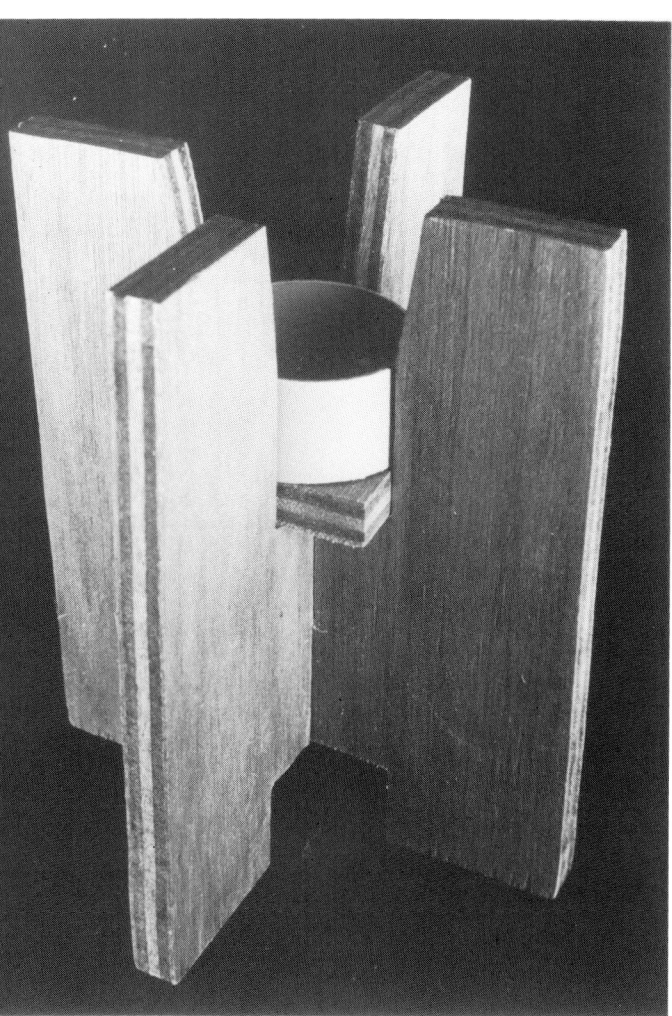

A Raising Block assembled

A Raising Block with a bed leg in place

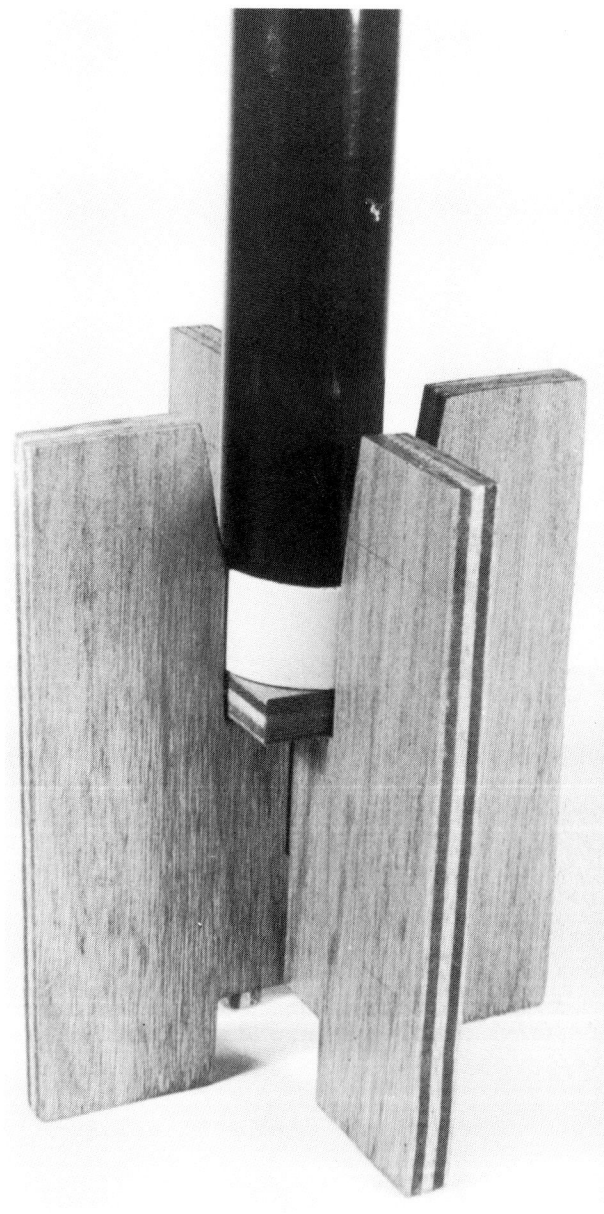

No glue or other fastening is required to hold these raising blocks together and they can be dismantled and packed flat for storage or transportation, which makes them particularly useful for nurses or therapists visiting patients in their own homes.

The uprights, of which eight are required for a full set, can be cut from 9 mm ($\frac{3}{8}$ in.) plywood, in the normal way. Some care should be exercised in cutting the interlocking vertical slots so that they fit snugly together, otherwise the blocks may wobble when assembled. The bearing blocks, of which four are needed for a set, can be provided easily by trimming offcuts from the uprights. As mentioned, the four 50 mm (2 in.) high locating rings are made by cutting them from a length of standard PVC pipe of 51 mm (2 in.) diameter.

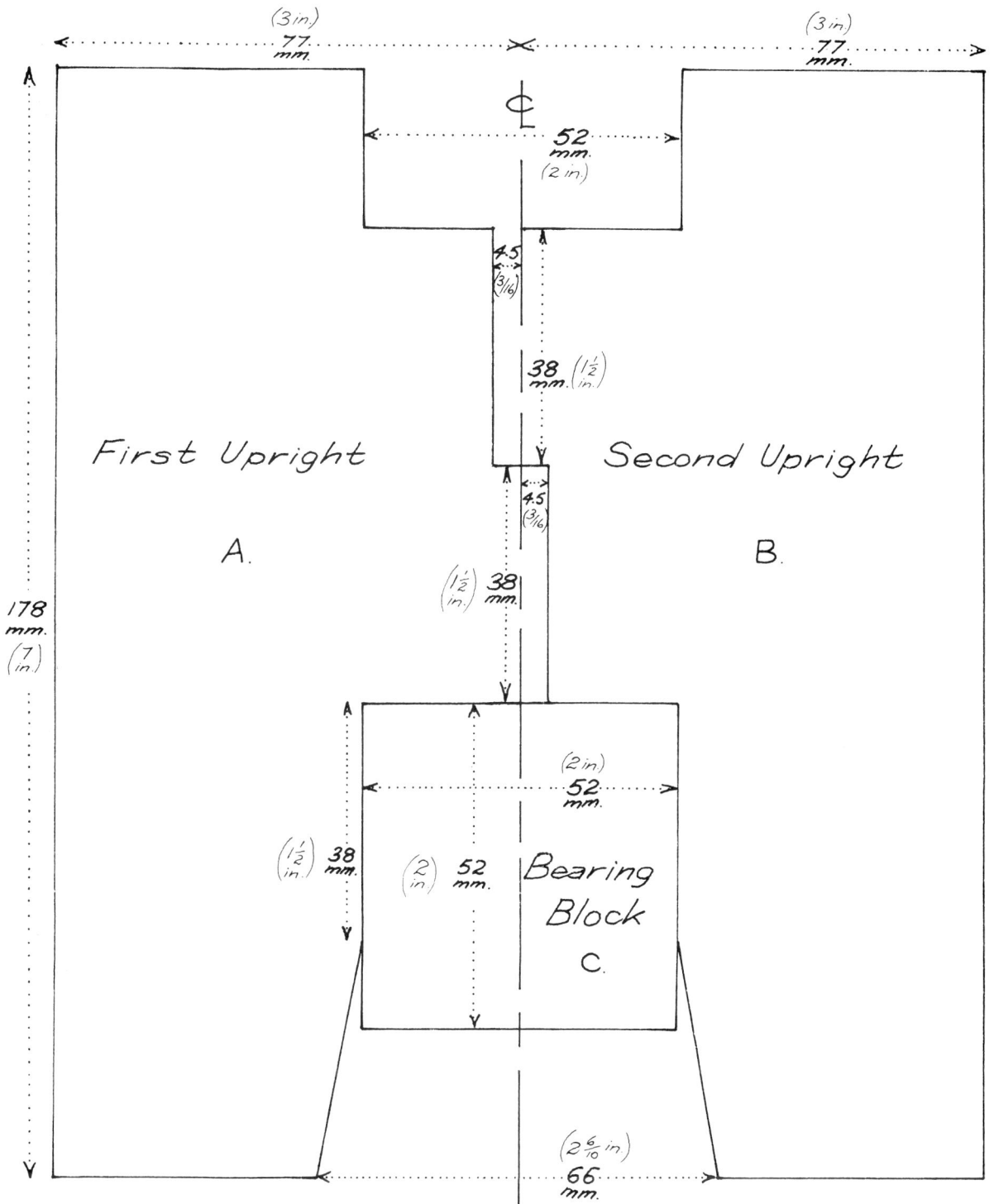

Reversible Dual Height Raising Block.

All pieces cut from 9mm. plywood. (3/8 in)

THE PAGE TURNER

This is a very simple aid, intended to enable pages of a book to be separated and turned by a person with limited reach or manual dexterity, or indeed with none at all, since it is possible to operate this device with one end held in the mouth. The rubber thimble, which is the vital component, can be bought for a very modest price from any stationer or office equipment retailer and is, of course, a valuable aid in its own right.

There are only four simple components, including the rubber thimble mentioned above, the others being a couple of wine bottle corks, a drugget pin and a straight piece of a wire coat hanger, about 300 mm (12 in.) long. A drugget pin is very similar to a good quality drawing pin, which could be used instead, but a drugget pin is preferred because it is longer.

One of the corks should be rounded off at one end, using a rasp or a knife, so that the rubber thimble can be fitted over it. The drugget pin is pushed into the side of the cork where it emerges from the thimble, leaving about 6 to 8 mm ($\frac{1}{4}$ to $\frac{5}{16}$ in.) of the pin protruding below the head. The two corks are then placed onto each end of the length of wire, the unmodified one serving as a handle.

Pages can be turned with the rubber thimble, either by pushing diagonally upward and inward from the right hand bottom corner of the page, or by pulling diagonally downward and inward from the right hand top corner. By rotating the device clockwise the edge of the drugget pin can be slipped in between pages to separate them, if necessary, as shown in the illustration.

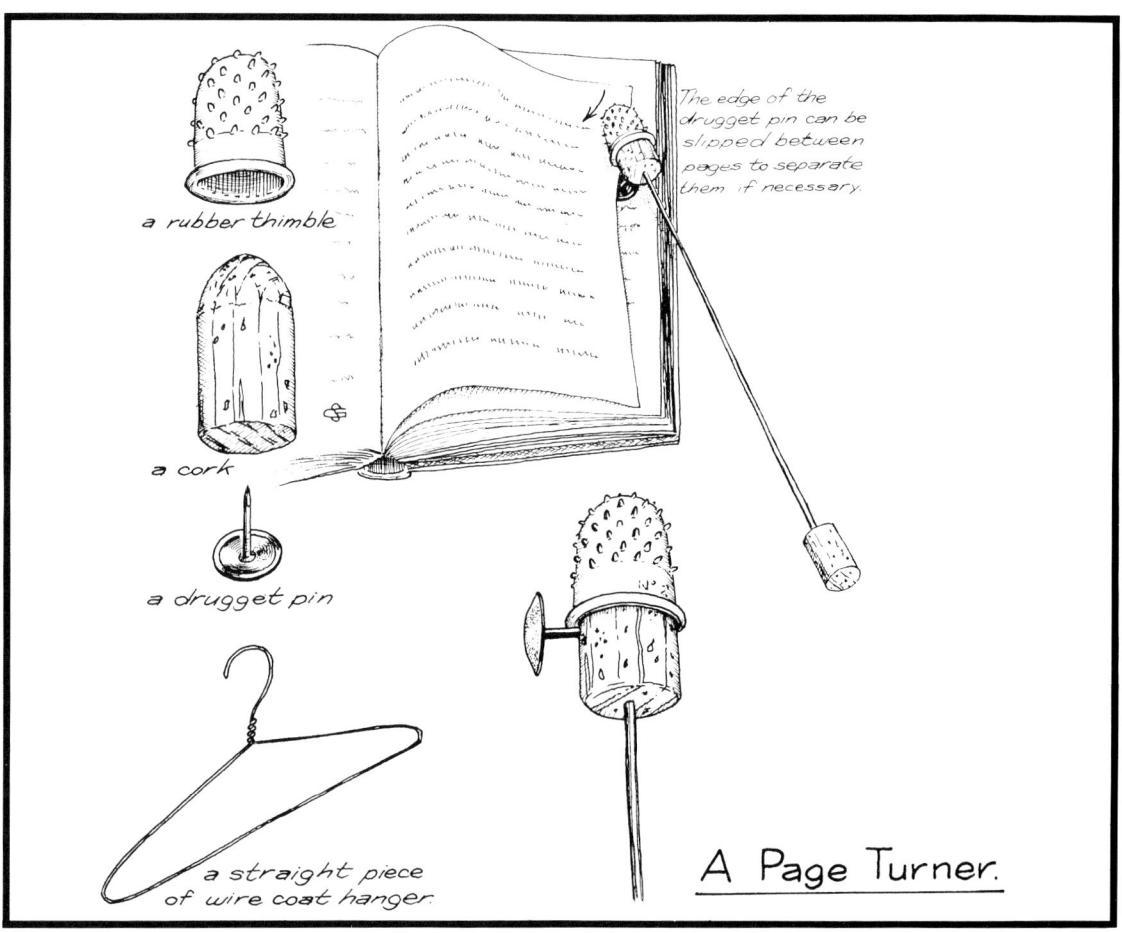

The edge of the drugget pin can be slipped between pages to separate them if necessary.

a rubber thimble

a cork

a drugget pin

a straight piece of wire coat hanger.

A Page Turner.

THE PAGE RESTRAINER

This is another very simple device and can be a great help to a handicapped reader, its purpose being to hold the pages of a book down so that they can be read easily, at the same time allowing the pages to be turned without difficulty. A reader who only has the use of one hand, for instance, can find it quite difficult to cope with a new book, or one that does not readily fall open. A reader who needs to use a Page Turner would find the use of a pair of Page Restrainers, placed one on each side of the book, a tremendous asset.

Page Restrainers cost very little and can be made very quickly, requiring only a standard Bulldog paper clip, about 50 mm (2 in.) wide, two pieces of fairly strong wire, such as that used in wire coat hangers, each piece about 150 mm (6 in.) long, a nut and bolt about 6 mm ($\frac{1}{4}$ in.) diameter and

as they act as bearings or pivot points, through which the second piece of wire rotates.

At the centre of the second piece of wire a curve is formed, which locates the second wire relative to the first, the curve being positioned between the bearing circles of the first wire (3). The two legs of the second wire are bent forward, spreading slightly outwards, as indicated by the approximate dimensions shown in (4), and the end of each is rolled into a small circle. These two small circles are the parts of the device which bear down upon the page of a book, the pressure being determined by the elastic band.

The wire assembly is bolted to the upper finger plate of the Bulldog clip, using the nut and bolt, which should pass through the hole normally provided in all such clips. One end of the elastic band is

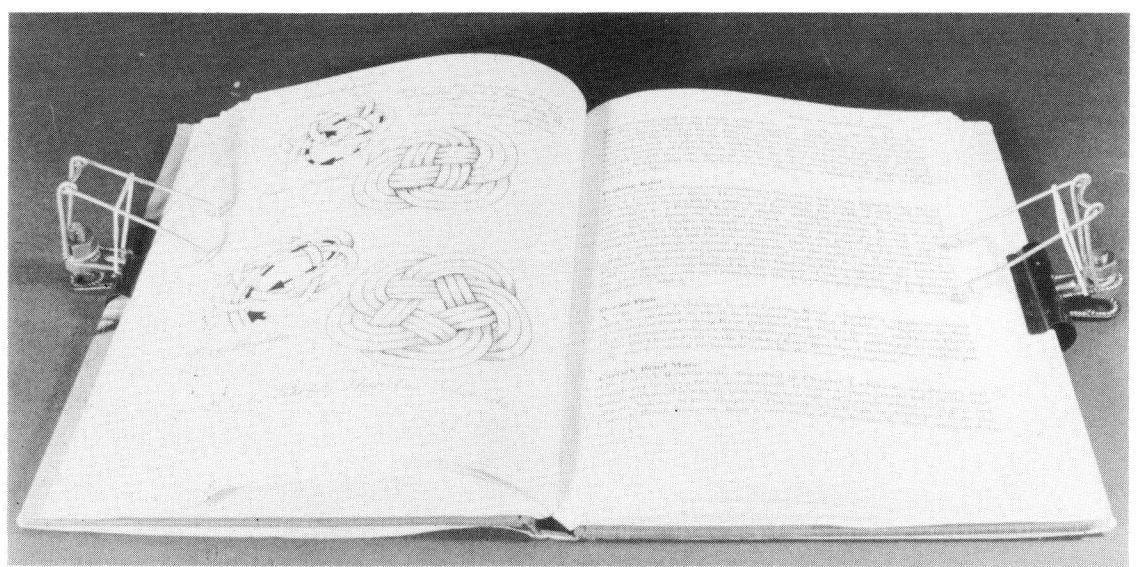

A pair of Page Restrainers fitted to the cover of a hardback book

12 mm ($\frac{1}{2}$ in.) long, and an ordinary elastic band about 40 mm ($1\frac{1}{2}$ in.) long.

Using a pair of pliers, preferably fairly pointed, the two pieces of wire are bent, as shown in the diagrams. Holding the first piece of wire about halfway along its length with the pair of pliers, make a circular loop just big enough to fit over the bolt (1); then bend each leg upward through a right angle, and roll the end of each (2) into a small circle, through which the second piece of wire can pass. These two small circles should be in line and parallel,

passed beneath the upper finger plate of the clip and behind the head of the bolt, while the other end passes over the two wire legs or fingers.

The Page Restrainer can be applied directly to a book with a hard cover, in which case the Bulldog clip is fastened to the edge of the cover and the wire fingers are lifted over the edge of the open pages, holding them down under the tension of the elastic band. In the case of a paperback book it is necessary to provide a semi-rigid surface beneath the pages, to which the Restrainer can be clipped. For the average

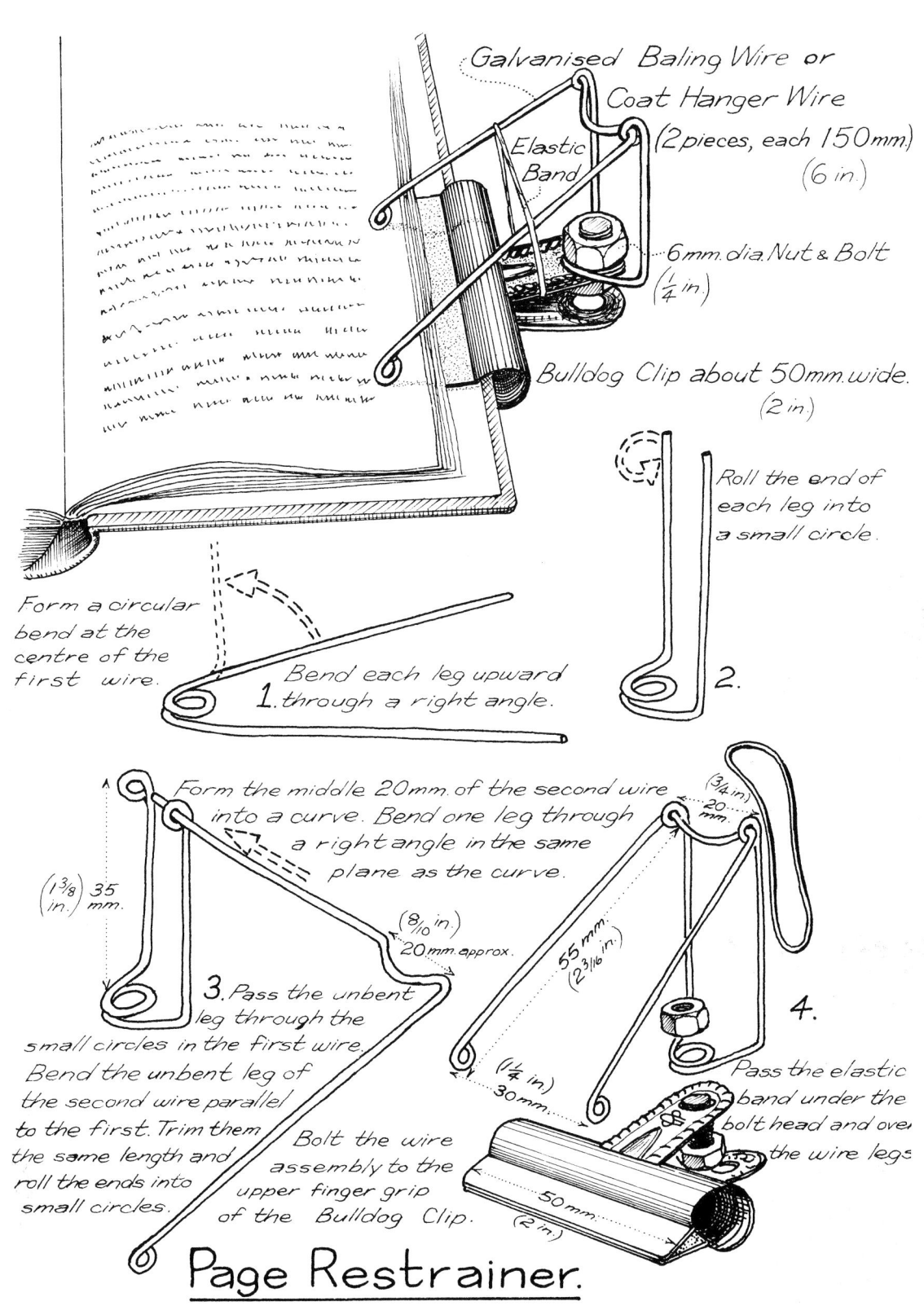

Galvanised Baling Wire or Coat Hanger Wire (2 pieces, each 150mm.) (6 in.)

Elastic Band

6mm. dia. Nut & Bolt ($\frac{1}{4}$ in.)

Bulldog Clip about 50mm. wide. (2 in.)

Roll the end of each leg into a small circle.

2.

Form a circular bend at the centre of the first wire.

Bend each leg upward
1. through a right angle.

Form the middle 20mm. of the second wire into a curve. Bend one leg through a right angle in the same plane as the curve.

($1\frac{3}{8}$ in.) 35 mm.

($\frac{8}{10}$ in.) 20 mm. approx.

3. Pass the unbent leg through the small circles in the first wire. Bend the unbent leg of the second wire parallel to the first. Trim them the same length and roll the ends into small circles.

Bolt the wire assembly to the upper finger grip of the Bulldog Clip.

($\frac{3}{4}$ in.) 20 mm.

55 mm. ($2\frac{3}{16}$ in.)

($\frac{1}{4}$ in.) 30 mm.

50 mm. (2 in.)

4.

Pass the elastic band under the bolt head and over the wire legs.

Page Restrainer.

22

paperback a piece of stiff cardboard, hardboard, thin plywood, plastic or metal sheet, measuring 180 mm (7 in.) from top to bottom and 230 mm (9 in.) from one side to the other is about right and any minor variations can be accommodated by the Restrainer. The semi-rigid board or sheet is placed beneath the open book and the Bulldog clip of the Restrainer is positioned so that it holds the cover of the book to the board, the wire fingers resting above the open page.

Providing that the elastic band is of about the right size and tension — and a little experimentation will soon find the optimum — the edge of a page can be slipped out from beneath the wire fingers of a Restrainer and back again without difficulty or risk of damage to the book. If a pair of Restrainers are placed one on each side of an open book the pages can be turned over, whilst constantly under contol, being slipped from one Restrainer to the other with no more than a finger tip (or a Page Turner) being used.

BOOK REST

This is a simple form of easel, on which an open book can be placed to rest on a table or other horizontal surface at a convenient angle for reading. The Book Rest has been designed so that, when fitted with Page Restrainers, it will hold a paperback book of average size in the most serviceable way. The Book Rest is big enough and sufficiently sturdy to hold large, heavy books if it is required to do so, and it has proved entirely satisfactory when used with the largest volume of a leather bound edition of the Encyclopaedia Brittanica. Page Restrainers can be attached to the cover of a hardback book, of course, so the size of the Book Rest relative to such books is less important than it is to paperbacks. One positive advantage of the small size and weight of the Book Rest is that it is convenient and unobtrusive to carry around.

Materials

A piece of ordinary hardboard or plywood about 3 mm ($\frac{1}{8}$ in.) thick, measuring 250 x 200 mm (10 x 8 in.) forms Part A (see diagram).

A piece of quarter round section wood about 15 mm ($\frac{5}{8}$ in.) radius and 250 mm (10 in.) long forms Part B.

A 252 mm (10 in.) length of 19 mm ($\frac{3}{4}$ in.) square section hardwood provides Part C and Parts D.

Part E is 60 mm ($2\frac{3}{8}$ in.) diameter hardwood dowelling.

Four No. 4 countersunk screws about 16 mm ($\frac{5}{8}$ in.) long and a little wood glue complete the requirements.

Construction

Part A—the edges of the Rest should be sanded smooth and the four counter sunk holes drilled in the positions shown in the drawing, with the countersink in the upper or smooth face of the board.

Part B—the Fiddle Is glued in position along the lower edge of Part A, with the radius facing outward.

Part C—support and Parts D—bearings Cut from the square section hardwood and drill a hole midway through the thickness of each in the position shown in the drawing to accept 8 mm ($\frac{5}{16}$ in.) diameter dowelling. The hole in the Support — Part

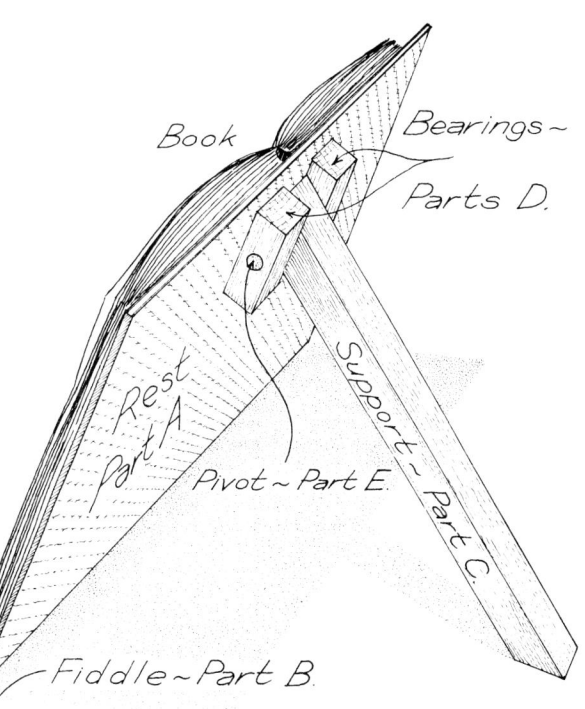

Book Rest.

Book

Bearings ~ Parts D.

Rest ~ Part A

Pivot ~ Part E

Support ~ Part C.

Fiddle ~ Part B.

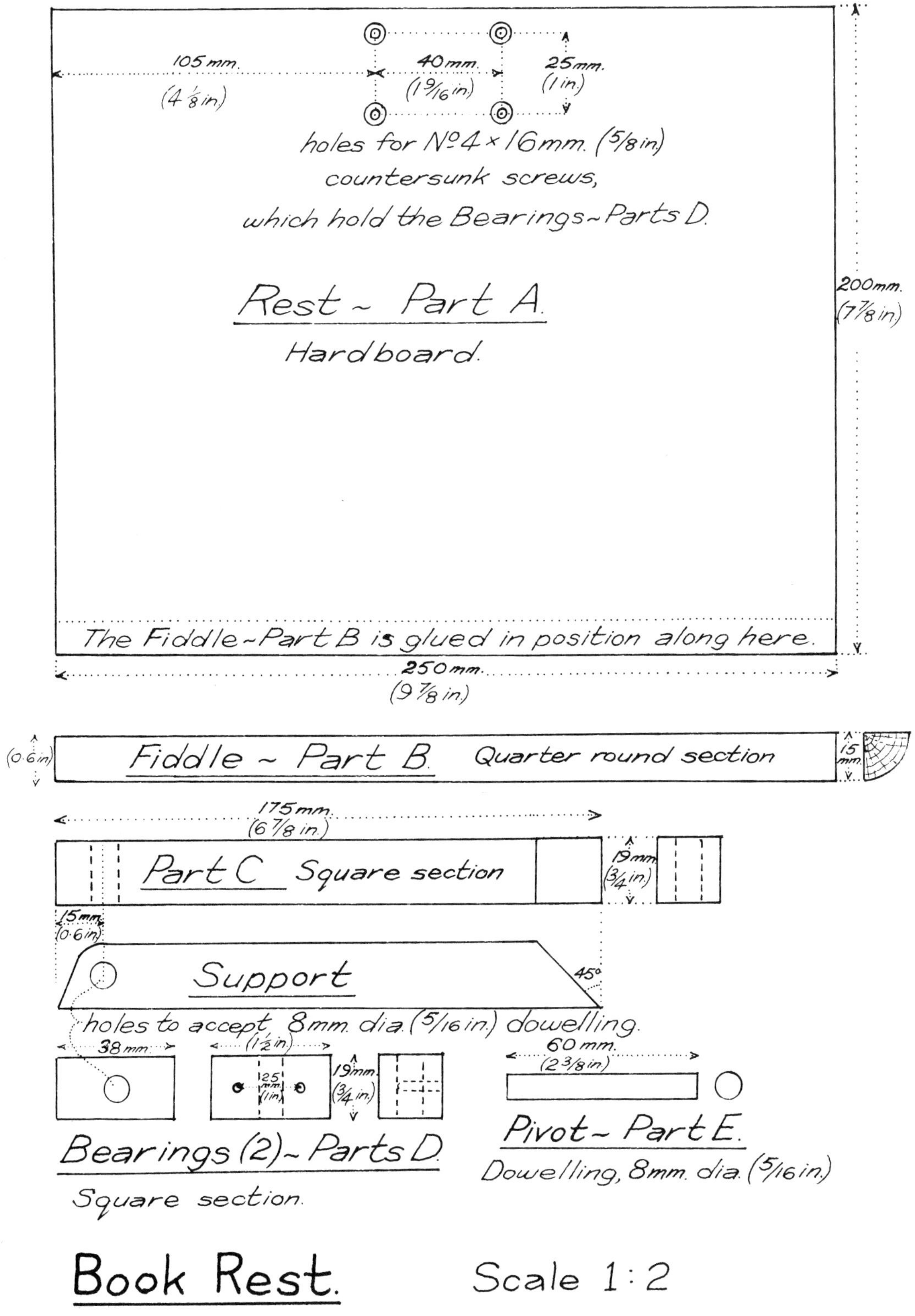

105 mm.
(4 $\frac{1}{8}$ in)

40 mm.
(1 $\frac{9}{16}$ in)

25 mm.
(1 in)

holes for N°4 × 16mm. (5/8 in)

countersunk screws,

which hold the Bearings~Parts D.

Rest ~ Part A.

Hardboard.

200mm.
(7 $\frac{7}{8}$ in)

The Fiddle~Part B is glued in position along here.

250 mm.
(9 $\frac{7}{8}$ in)

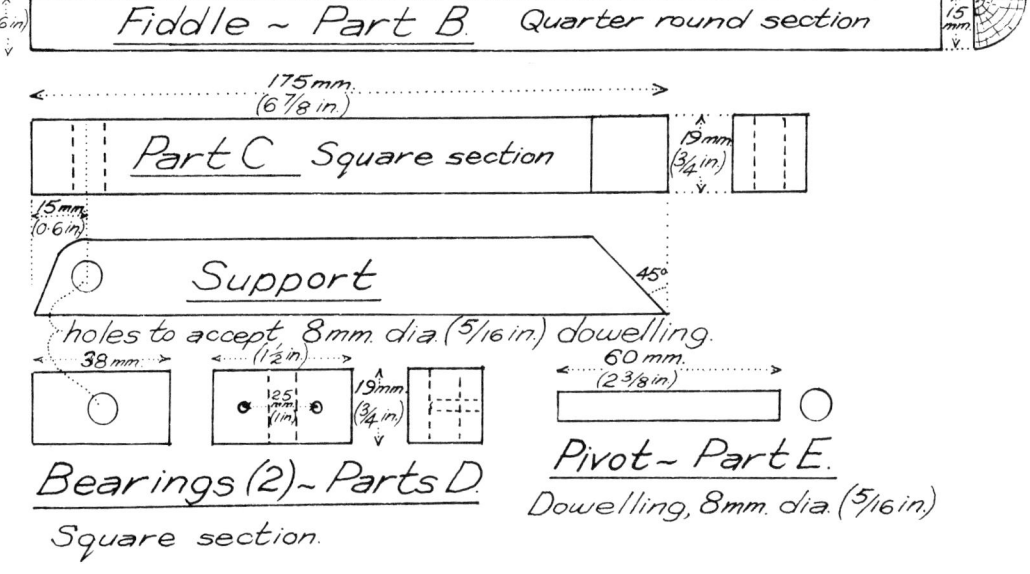

(0·6 in)

Fiddle ~ Part B.   Quarter round section

15 mm

175 mm.
(6 $\frac{7}{8}$ in)

Part C   Square section

19 mm
(3/4 in)

15 mm
(0·6 in)

Support

45°

holes to accept 8mm. dia. (5/16 in.) dowelling.

38 mm

(1 $\frac{1}{2}$ in)

12·5 mm (1 in)

19 mm
(3/4 in.)

60 mm.
(2 $\frac{3}{8}$ in)

Bearings (2) ~ Parts D.

Square section.

Pivot ~ Part E.

Dowelling, 8mm. dia. (5/16 in.)

Book Rest.   Scale 1:2

C — should be very slightly larger than the others so that the Pivot will move freely in it.

Part C Shape the Support at both ends as shown in the drawing, using a saw, rasp and glasspaper.

Part E—the Pivot Glue one end into position through one Bearing — Part D — its end flush with the hole.

Part E Pass the free end of the Pivot through the hole in the Support — Part C — and then into the hole in the second Bearing — Part D. The Support should swing quite freely on the Pivot with the Bearings held fixed.

The assembly of Support, Bearings and Pivot can now be offered up to the back of the Rest — Part A — so that the positions of the lead holes for the screws can be marked on the Bearings. The lead holes are then drilled into the Bearings and they can be screwed onto the back of the Rest — Part A — making sure that the chamfers of the Support — Part C — face inward.

The Book Rest may be varnished or painted but this is not essential.

The Book Rest with Page Restrainers in place

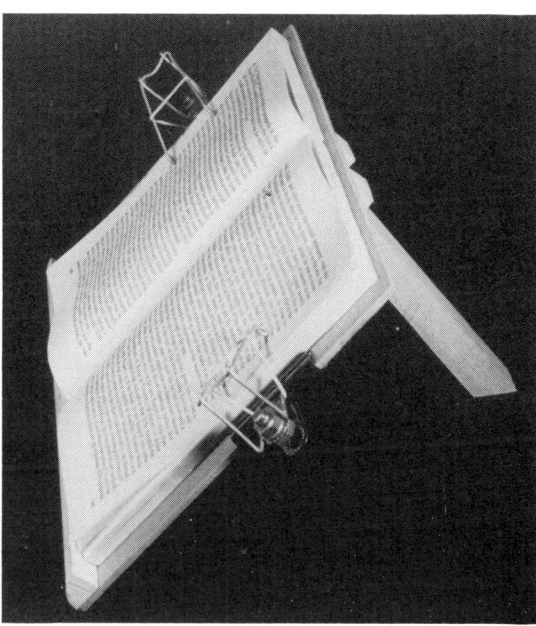

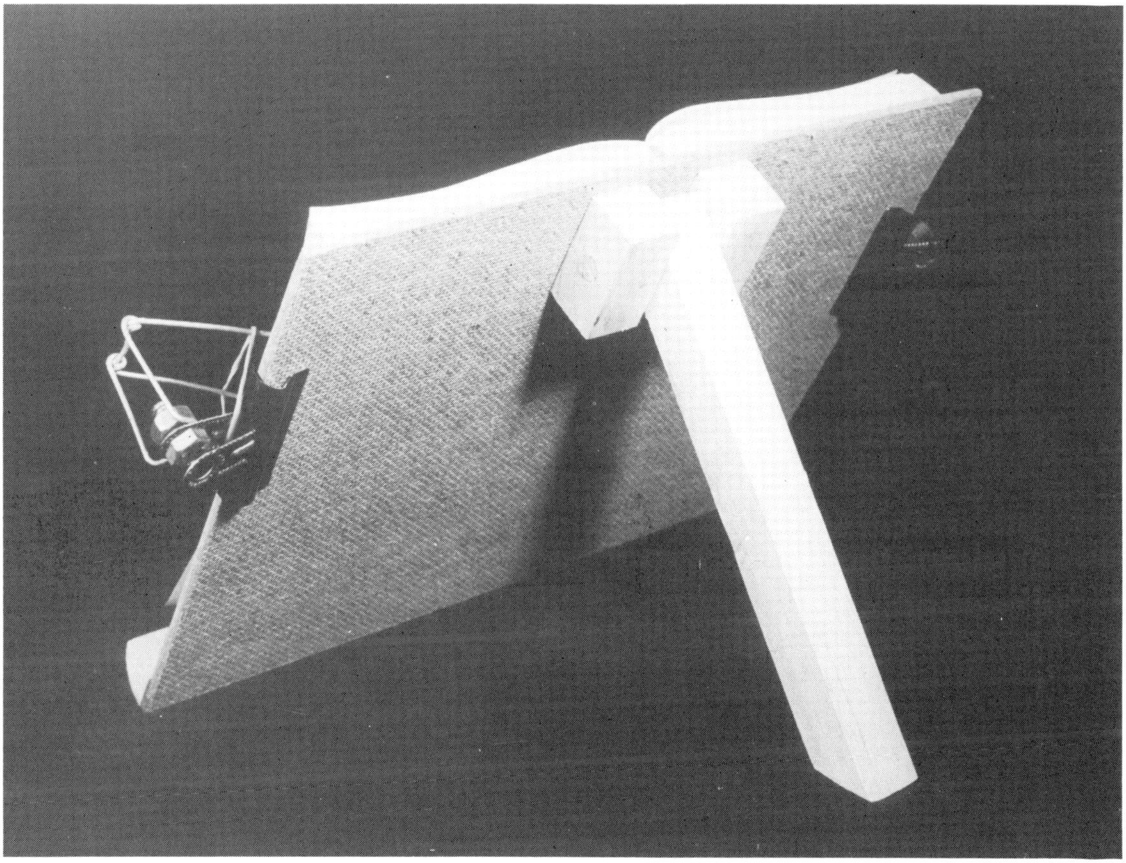

The Book Rest viewed from the back

THE GRIPPER

The Gripper is a very simple implement to make and can be an invaluable aid to anyone with weakened or disabled hands. Its purpose is to grip screw lids securely, for both opening and closing, but it may also be used to open and close taps and valves. It will hold any size of circular cap between a minimum diameter of 19 mm ($\frac{3}{4}$ in.) and a maximum diameter of 76 mm (3 in.), which latitude includes most household containers, from a coffee or pickle jar to a sauce bottle.

The elastic band between parts A and C (see diagram) is not essential, and the Gripper can be operated quite well without it, but it is convenient sometimes to be able to leave the Gripper in place for a few minutes, and the elastic band exerts sufficient tension between the jaws to provide this facility.

Construction

Parts A and C are cut to shape from 9 mm ($\frac{3}{8}$ in.) plywood using a coping saw or jigsaw and the 6 mm ($\frac{1}{4}$ in.) bolt hole is drilled in Part C.

Part B of which two are required, are cut from 4 mm ($\frac{3}{16}$ in.) plywood and the 6 mm ($\frac{1}{4}$ in.) bolt holes are drilled.

Assembly

The two parts B are glued overlapping the outer faces of Part A as shown in the diagram. Drill pilot holes and countersink so as to reinforce this glued 'sandwich' with the three No. 6 screws, entering two from one side and one from the other. If their points project through the wood, file them down flush. Glue a 140 mm ($5\frac{1}{2}$ in.) strip of rubber on the inner face of Part A and a 70 mm ($2\frac{3}{4}$ in.) strip on the inner face of Part C, as shown in the diagrams, and secure these strips with two or three tacks. Place Part C between the two Parts B, align the bolt holes and enter the bolt; position the lock washer beneath the nut and screw it up hand tight, so that the arms of the Gripper open and close freely. Screw the two eyes into the ends of Parts A and C and place the elastic band between them.

Materials

A small piece of 4 mm ($\frac{3}{16}$ in.) plywood about 75 mm (3 in.) square.

A piece of 9 mm ($\frac{3}{8}$ in.) plywood about 150 x 160 mm (6 x $6\frac{3}{8}$ in.). The thickness of the plywood is not critical but the stated sizes are about optimum.

3 No. 6 x 18 mm (or $\frac{5}{8}$ in.) countersunk screws.

1 round or flat head bolt 6 mm ($\frac{1}{4}$ in.) x 25 mm (1 in.) with lock washer and nut.

A strip of rubber from an old tyre inner tube 9 mm x 210 mm ($\frac{3}{8}$ x $8\frac{1}{4}$ in.).

A few tacks and a little impact adhesive.

2 small screw eyes and one elastic band 35 mm ($1\frac{3}{8}$ in.) unstretched.

Using the Gripper

It is helpful to mark the Gripper on the appropriate side with the word 'OPEN', so that the user knows that when that side is uppermost the action of the Gripper will open a lid. Conversely, when the word 'OPEN' is facing downward and not visible, the Gripper will close a lid.

To open a large diameter lid, the point of the V in Part A may be placed against the user's chest while the Gripper's jaws are opened sufficiently to enclose the lid. Relatively little effort is needed to move the most stubborn lid with this device and it can be useful in any home, regardless of disablement.

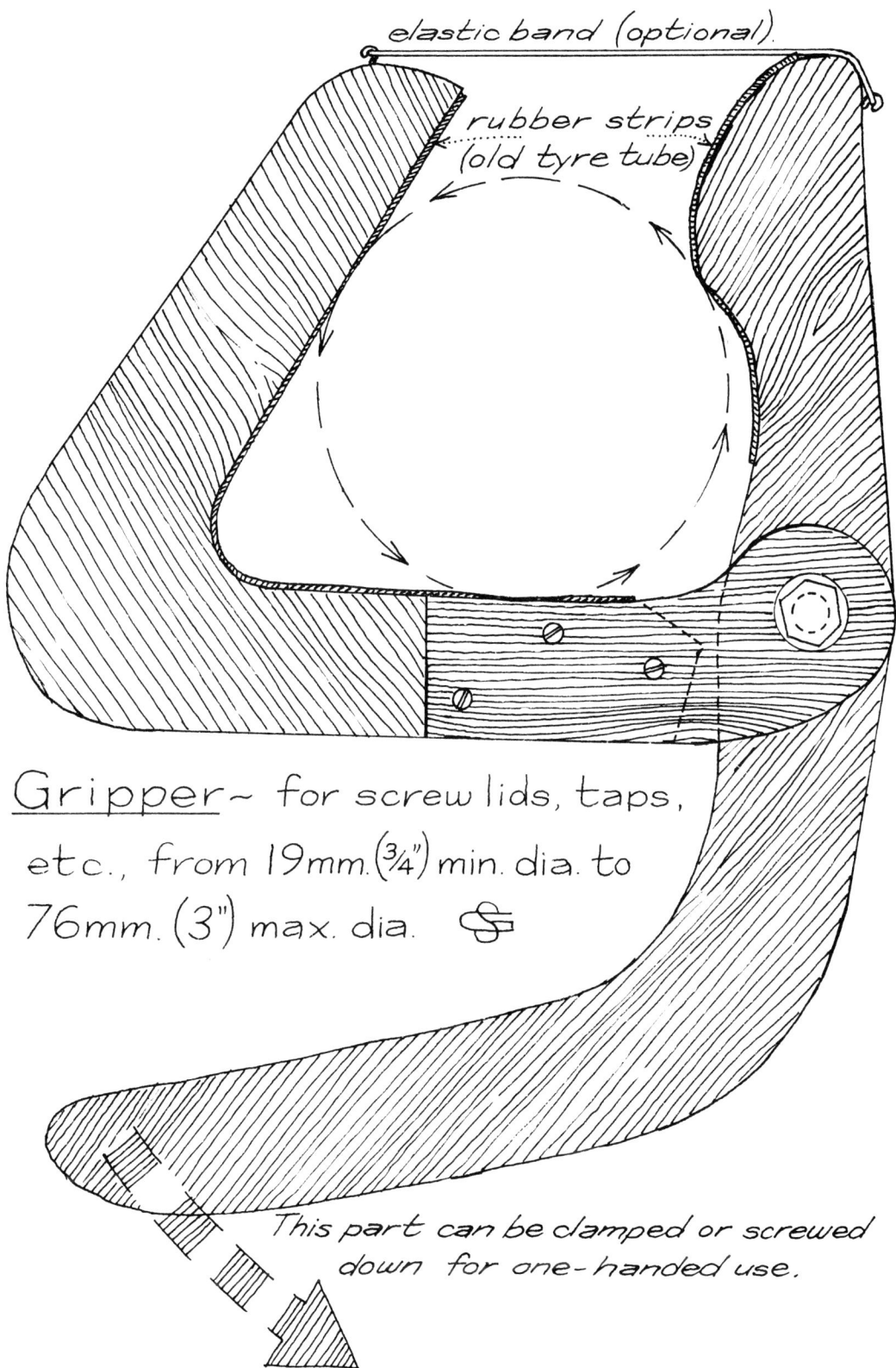

elastic band (optional).

rubber strips
(old tyre tube)

Gripper~ for screw lids, taps,
etc., from 19mm.(¾") min. dia. to
76mm. (3") max. dia.

This part can be clamped or screwed
down for one-handed use.

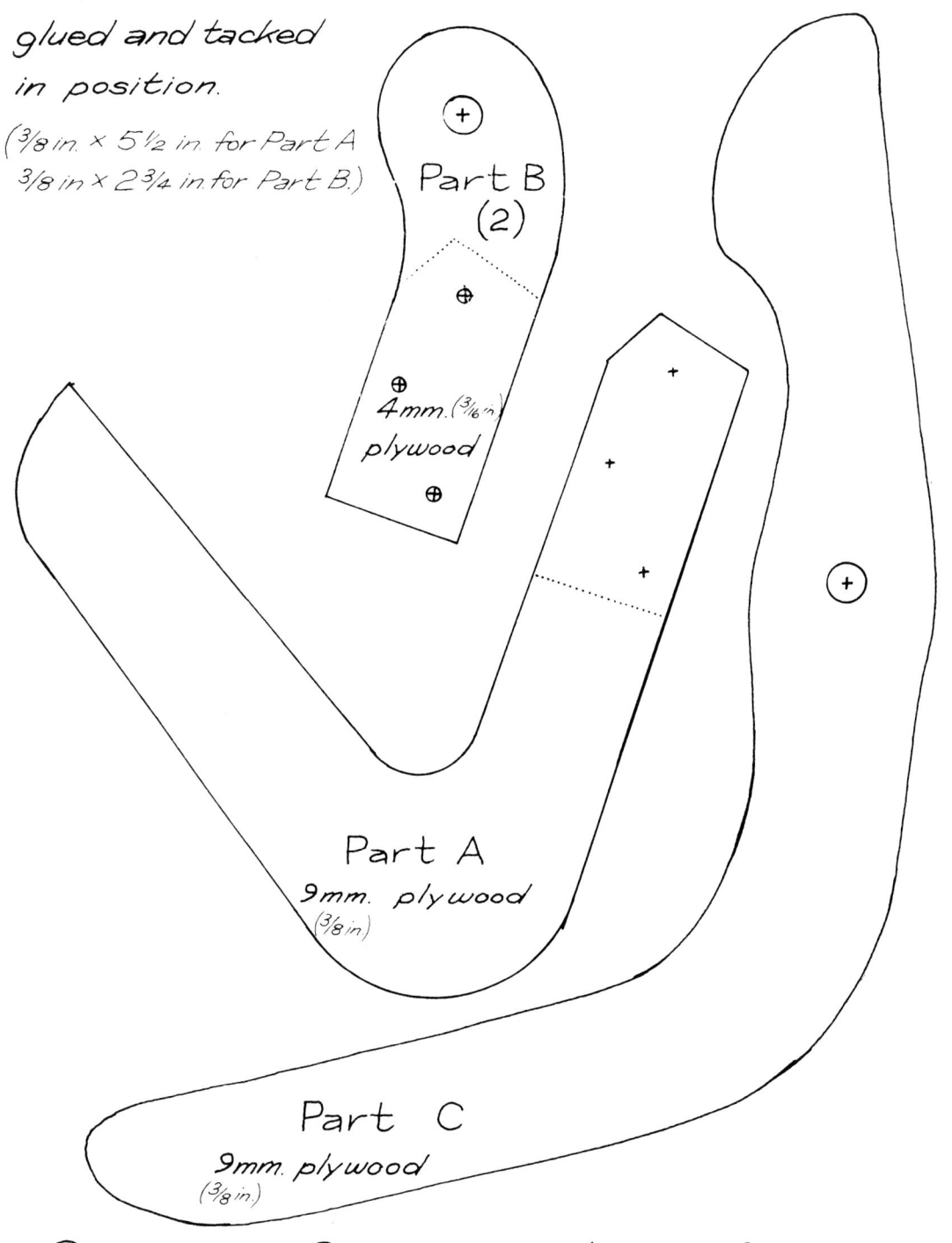

The Gripper's jaws are faced with rubber strips, 9 × 140 mm. for Part A, 9 × 70 mm. for Part C, glued and tacked in position.

(3/8 in. × 5½ in. for Part A
3/8 in × 2¾ in. for Part B.)

Part B
(2)

4mm. (3/16 in.)
plywood

Part A
9mm. plywood
(3/8 in.)

Part C
9mm. plywood
(3/8 in.)

Gripper Components.

Part A
Part B
Part C
Gripper

The Gripper in use

OPEN

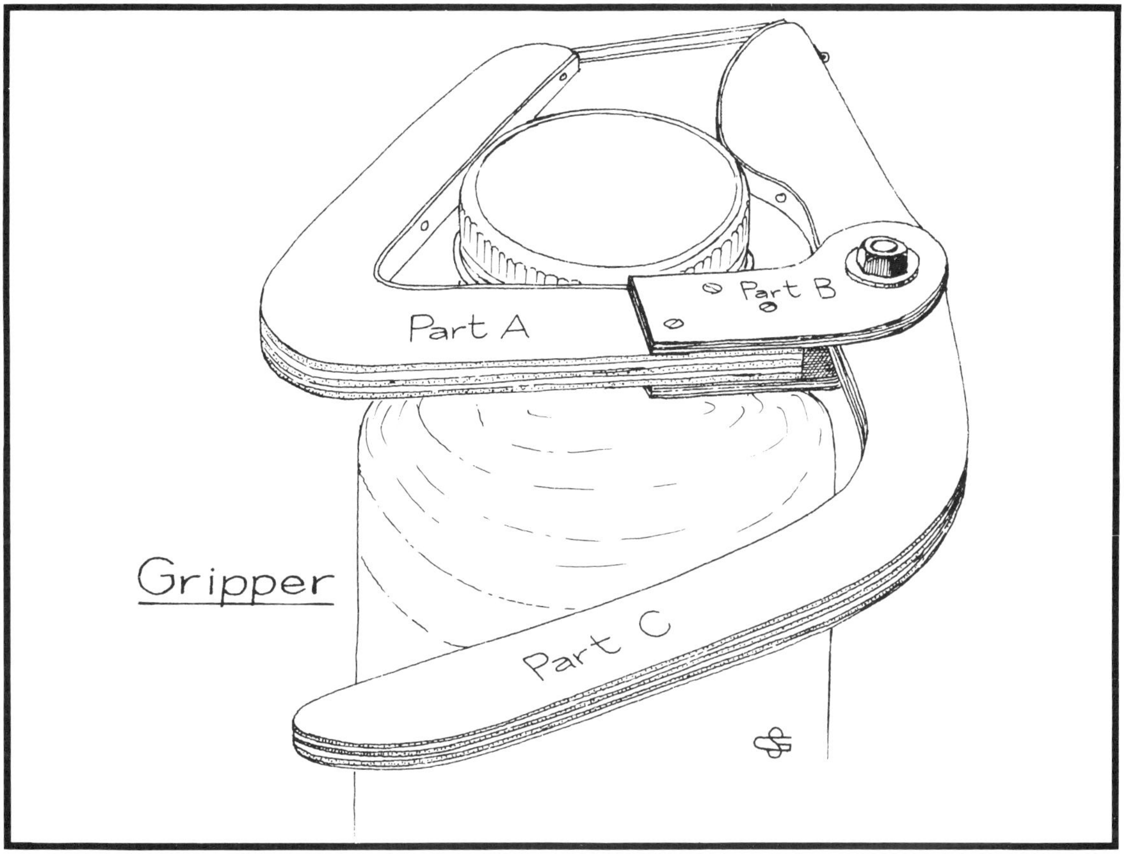

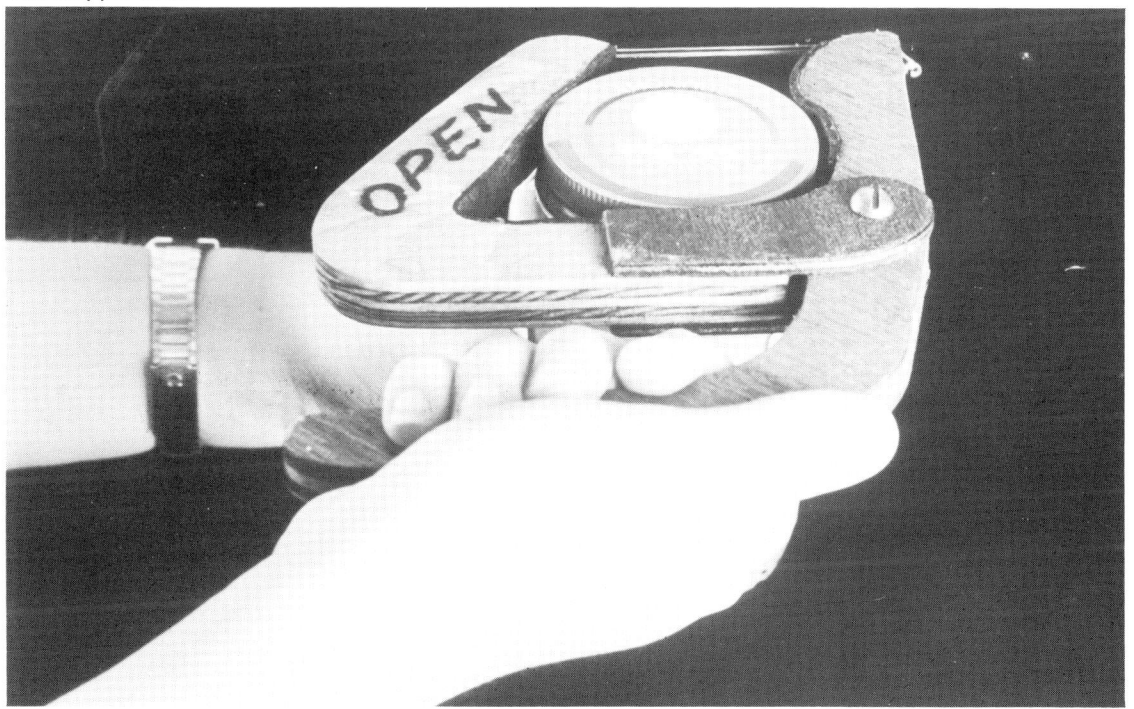

SPLIT SPIRALS

This is a most useful aid for innumerable purposes, just a few of which have been illustrated. Such spirals can be cut from any size of flexible tube to fit an unlimited range of tools. The two most appropriate and readily available of suitable tubes are ordinary garden hose and the type of heavy rubber pipe which is sold for use on portable gas appliances, in caravans and boats.

Note that the spiral can be cut in either of two directions, and one direction may be more appropriate than the other, depending upon the intended purpose. Different users have different preferences in this respect, and it is not merely a matter of which hand is being used, as one might expect. Note also that the central split between the upper and lower curls of the spiral is deliberately widened to make the opening of the spiral easier.

It is worth bearing in mind that a flexible spiral of this type will hold a range of objects of different dimensions equally well. A spiral of garden hose, for instance, will hold a fountain pen, a tube of paint, a ruler or a penknife to equally good effect. Split spirals can be screwed or bolted to almost anything

to provide a cheap and effective alternative to spring clips for storing tools. Bolted to a half section of plastic drainpipe, which comfortably fits in the hand, a split spiral will provide a means by which a hand disabled by arthritis, for instance, may hold cutlery, a pencil, toothbrush or knitting needle firmly positioned, yet easily removed or adjusted.

Probably the best tool to use for cutting these spirals is a razor saw of the kind used by model makers, but a sharp craft knife or junior hacksaw can be almost as effective.

It is advisable to mark out the cutting line with a chinagraph pencil or felt tip pen before attempting to cut, as it is not easy to judge the line accurately by eye and a little easily-adjusted experimentation with the pencil will save wasted time and temper, as well as tube. Remember to cut along the line with the cutting edge facing, as far as possible, directly into the centre of the tube, which therefore must be rotated gradually and steadily throughout the cutting process. This explanation probably makes the procedure sound much more complicated than it really is and a trial spiral or two will soon develop the technique.

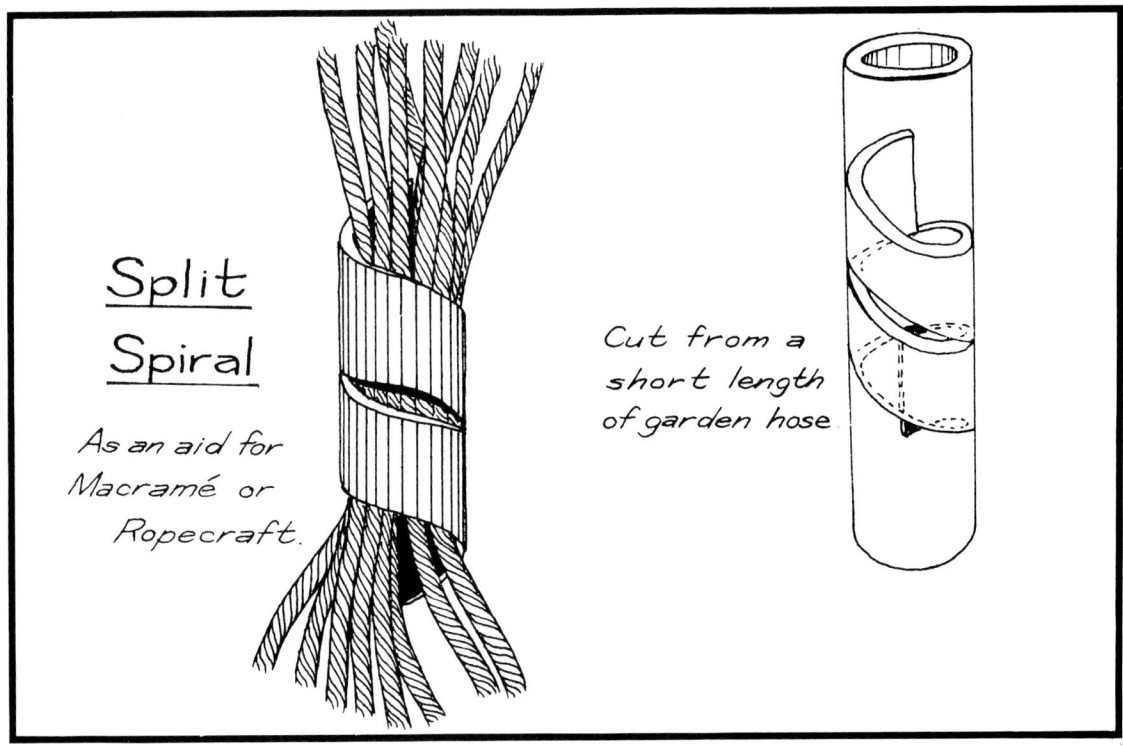

Split
Spiral

As an aid for
Macramé or
Ropecraft.

Cut from a
short length
of garden hose

A Split Spiral cut from a piece of heavy rubber gas pipe bolted to a halved section of 51mm.(2") p.v.c. drainpipe to make a holding aid for disabled hands.

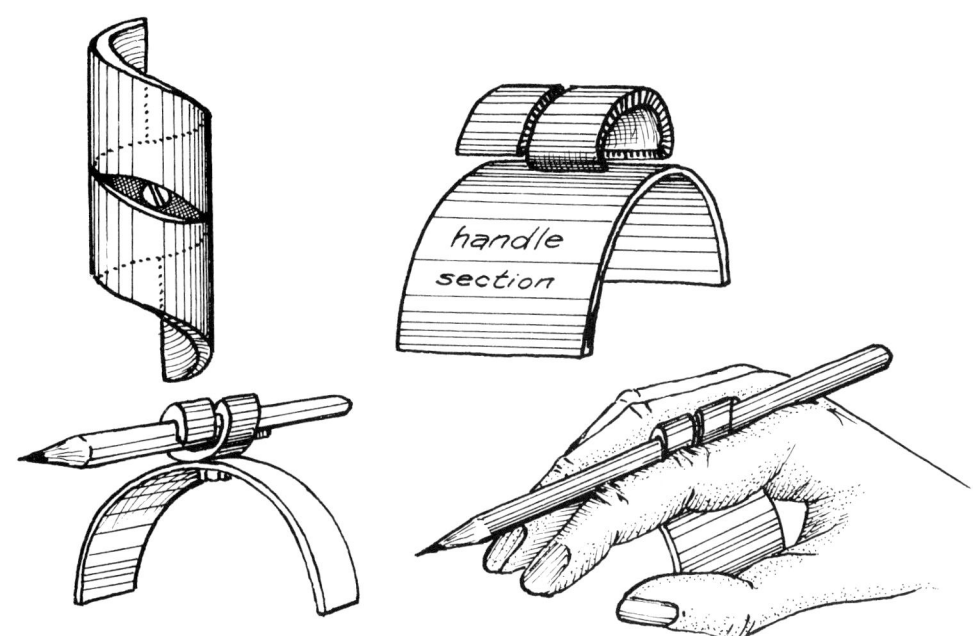

The Spiral of this device will adjust itself to hold many everyday tools, including cutlery, toothbrush, lipstick etc. Other sizes of tube for both Spiral and Handle may be used to suit particular purposes or disabilities.

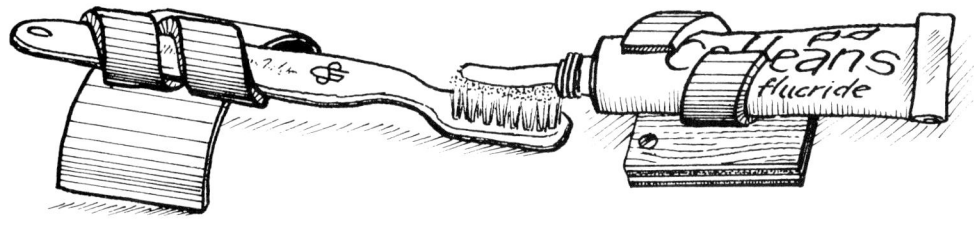

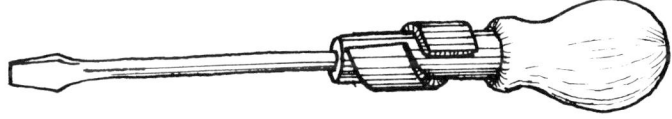

The Split Spiral~ all purpose aid.

BUCKLED SPIRALS

This is another use of the split spiral, two of which are here either riveted or bolted to a short length — 76 to 90 mm (3 to $3\frac{1}{2}$in.) — of PVC guttering about 80 mm ($3\frac{1}{8}$ in.) wide. If several such aids are required, an alternative rather stronger than guttering can be produced by cutting a piece of 101 mm (4 in.) diameter PVC pipe into three sections lengthwise.

The piece of guttering or pipe section is slotted, as shown in the drawing, by drilling a hole at each end of each slot and then cutting between the two holes with a coping saw. The slots form the piece of guttering or pipe section into a curved buckle, through which, on one side, a 450 mm (18 in.) mm length of 50 mm (2 in.) wide webbing can be adjusted and, on the other side, a loop of the webbing can be attached. The loop of webbing may be sewn in place, but if instead it is formed by a short length of Velcro fastening having been sewn across the webbing, as shown in the drawing, the device can be rapidly and easily secured in position or removed.

This aid was designed for use around the forearm of a man who had lost one hand, and enabled him to hold writing instruments, eating utensils· and tools. The two spirals might conveniently be made from two different sizes of tube, to increase the range of tools capable of being held. The spirals can be turned to any desired angle. Buckled Spirals can be attached to almost anything, of course; the arm of a chair or wheel chair for instance, to hold a knitting needle or crochet hook.

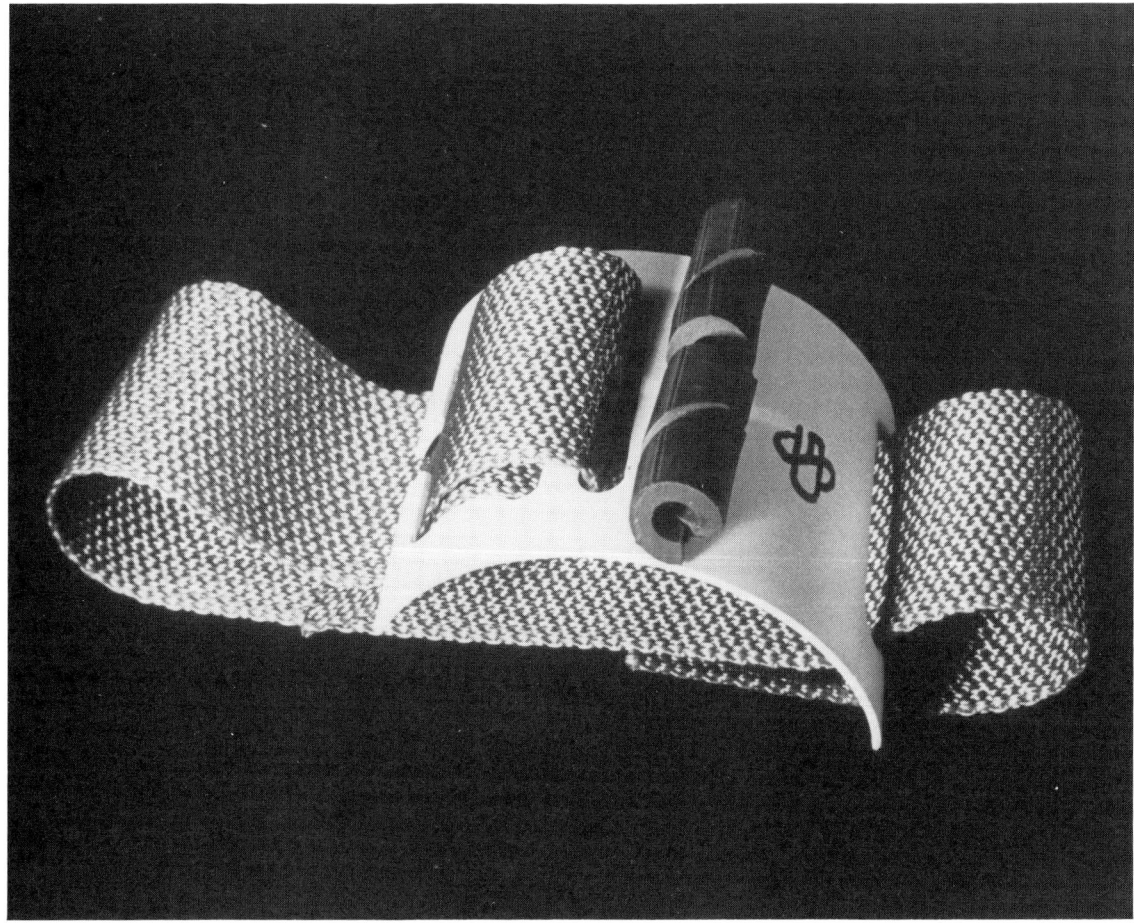

Gas pipe spirals fastened to a guttering buckle by pop rivets

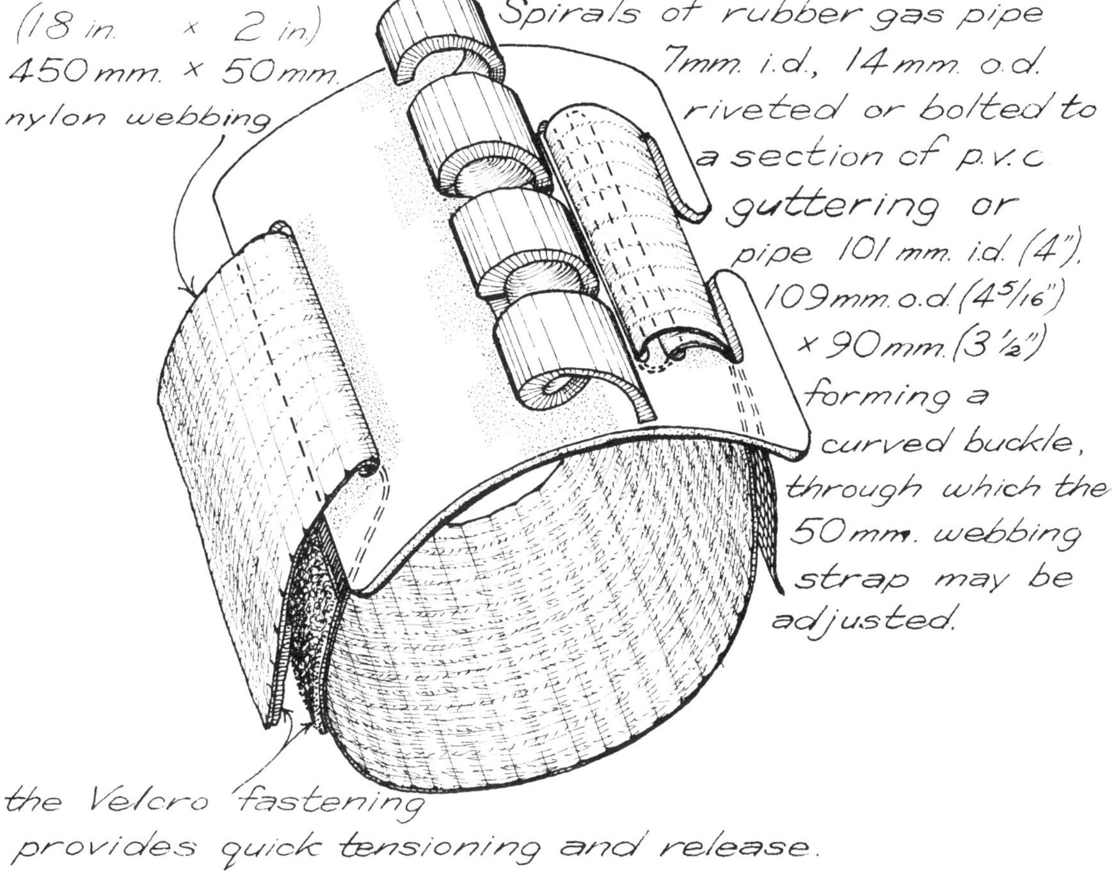

(18 in. × 2 in.)
450 mm. × 50 mm.
nylon webbing

Spirals of rubber gas pipe
7mm. i.d., 14mm. o.d.
riveted or bolted to
a section of p.v.c
guttering or
pipe 101 mm. i.d. (4"),
109mm.o.d (4⁵⁄₁₆")
× 90mm.(3½")
forming a
curved buckle,
through which the
50 mm. webbing
strap may be
adjusted.

the Velcro fastening
provides quick tensioning and release.

Buckled Spiral.

For strapping to a limb
or the arm of a chair.

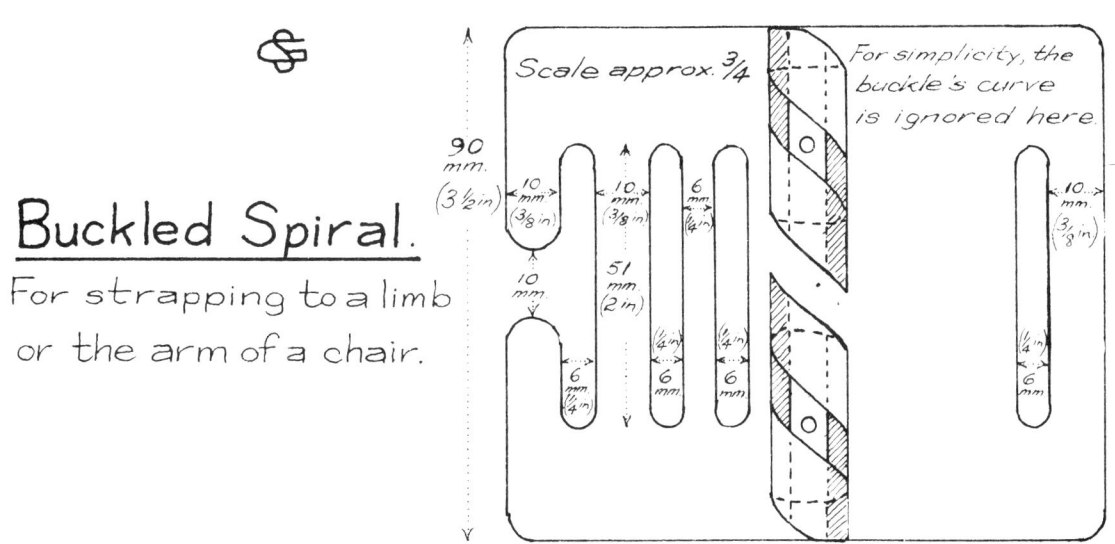

Scale approx. ³⁄₄

For simplicity, the
buckle's curve
is ignored here.

90
mm.
(3½in)

10
mm
(3⁄8in)

10.
mm
(3⁄8in)

6
mm
(¼in)

10
mm

51
mm
(2in)

6
mm
(¼in)

6
mm
(¼in)

6
mm
(¼in)

10..
mm
(3⁄8in)

¼in

6
mm

TUBULAR BUCKLE

The Tubular Buckle illustrated is made from a 76 mm (3 in.) length of PVC water pipe, having an outside diameter of 66 mm (2.6 in.) and wall thickness of 2.5 mm ($\frac{1}{8}$ in.), but such buckles may be made from plastic or metal tube of almost any convenient size, providing only that there is room for the slots. Similarly, the webbing specified in the drawing is 51 mm (2 in.) wide, but equally effective buckles may be produced to suit webbing of a smaller or larger width.

Notice that a tubular buckle of the kind illustrated can be used in two ways. As shown in (2) it is hooked on to a rail; it can be used equally well to hook on to a shelf or ledge fitted with beading, an angle iron or frame surrounding a bed or chair seat. The strength of the buckle used as a hook in this way is limited by the strength of the tubing, and thin walled plastic tube could be pulled off quite easily. Nevertheless, such buckle/hooks can be most useful in some circumstances.

The second method of use, as shown in (3), offers much greater security, because the webbing and buckle together completely surround the rail. This method can be used only when it is possible to completely encircle the rail.

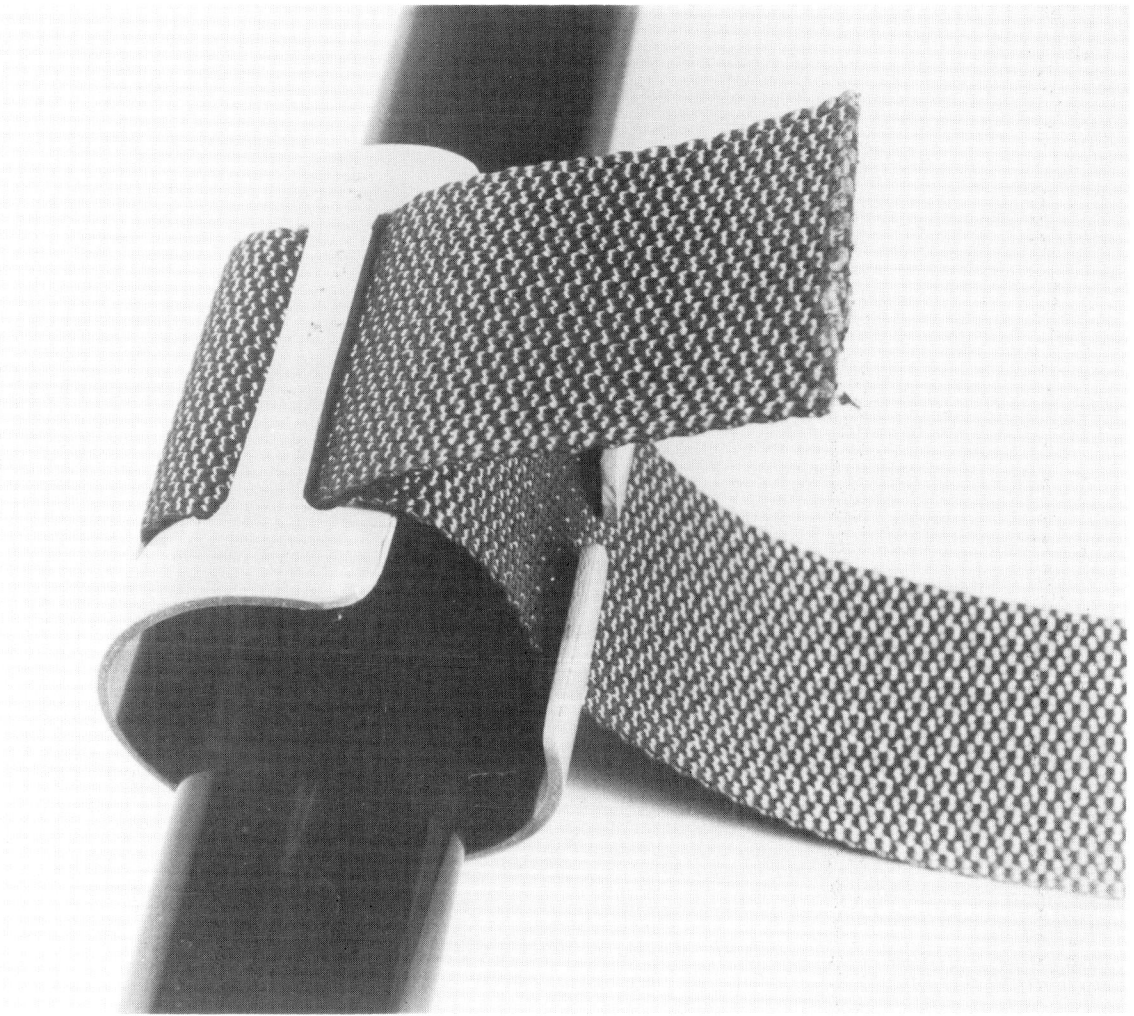

A Tubular Buckle around a bar

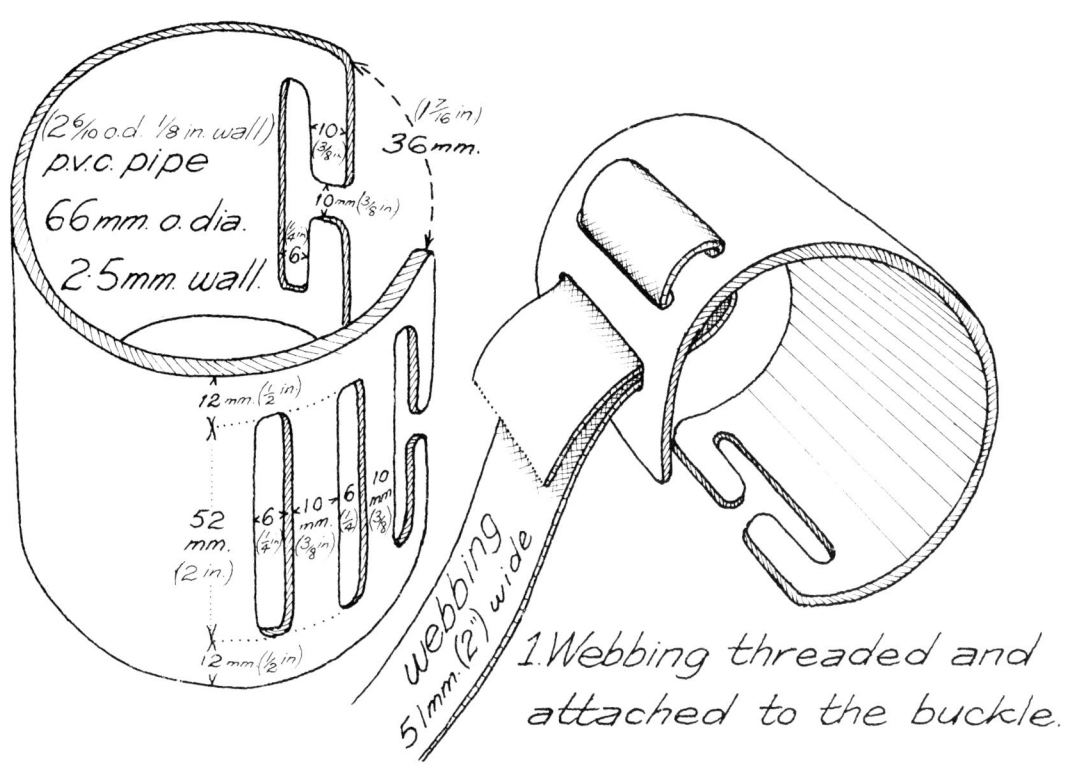

(2⁹⁄₁₀ o.d. ⅛ in. wall)
p.v.c. pipe
66mm. o.dia.
2·5mm. wall.

10 × (³⁄₈in.) (1⁷⁄₁₆ in.) 36mm.

10mm(³⁄₈ in)

¼in 6″

12mm.(½ in.)

52 mm. (2 in.)

6 (¼in.) 10mm.(³⁄₈in.) 6 (¼) 10mm. ³⁄₈

12mm.(½ in.)

webbing 51mm. (2″) wide

1. Webbing threaded and attached to the buckle.

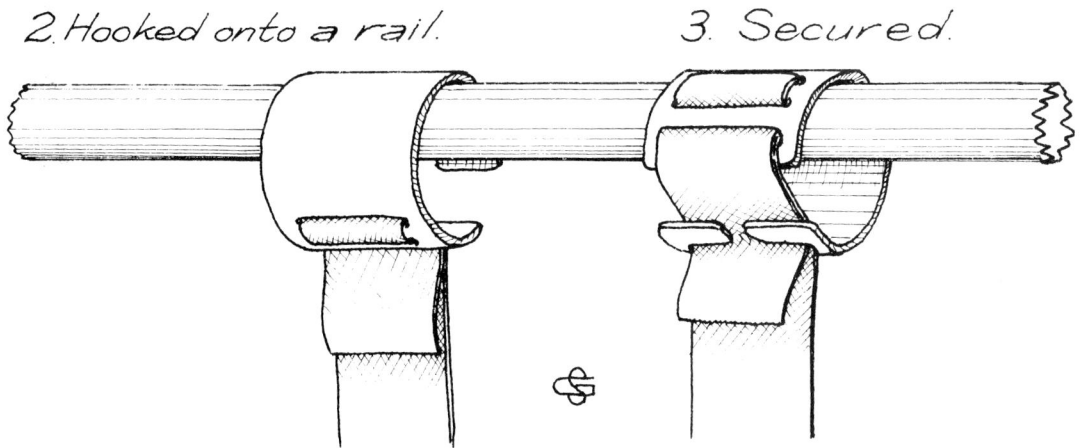

2. Hooked onto a rail.

3. Secured.

A Tubular Buckle.

To attach Webbing to a Rail or Bar

SHOE HORN

There can be few people who are unaware of the use of a shoe horn, for every shop retailing shoes provides them for helping customers ease new shoes onto their feet. A shoe horn can be an asset to anyone, but to many handicapped people it is an indispensible necessity. A shoe horn with an extended handle can be a great boon to anyone who finds it difficult to bend down. The shoe horn illustrated here is made from a short piece of plastic guttering, the width of which will comfortably yield two such shoe horns side by side, as shown in the diagram.

Materials

160 x 78 mm ($6\frac{1}{4}$ x $3\frac{1}{16}$ in.) of PVC guttering.

500 x 12 mm (20 x $\frac{1}{2}$ in.) dowelling or square section hardwood.

2 round head screws No. 4 or No. 6.

A short length of twine, wire, ribbon or tape for the hanging loop.

Construction

Trace a paper template from the pattern provided and draw the shape on the plastic guttering. Cut out the shape, using a coping saw, fretsaw or piercing saw; alternatively it is possible with care to cut this material successfully with the type of snips designed to cut thin sheet metal. Clean up the cut edges with glass paper and drill the screw holes. The shoe horn now can be screwed to one end of the length of dowelling or square section hardwood, which forms an extended handle, through which a hole is drilled at the other end for the hanging loop.

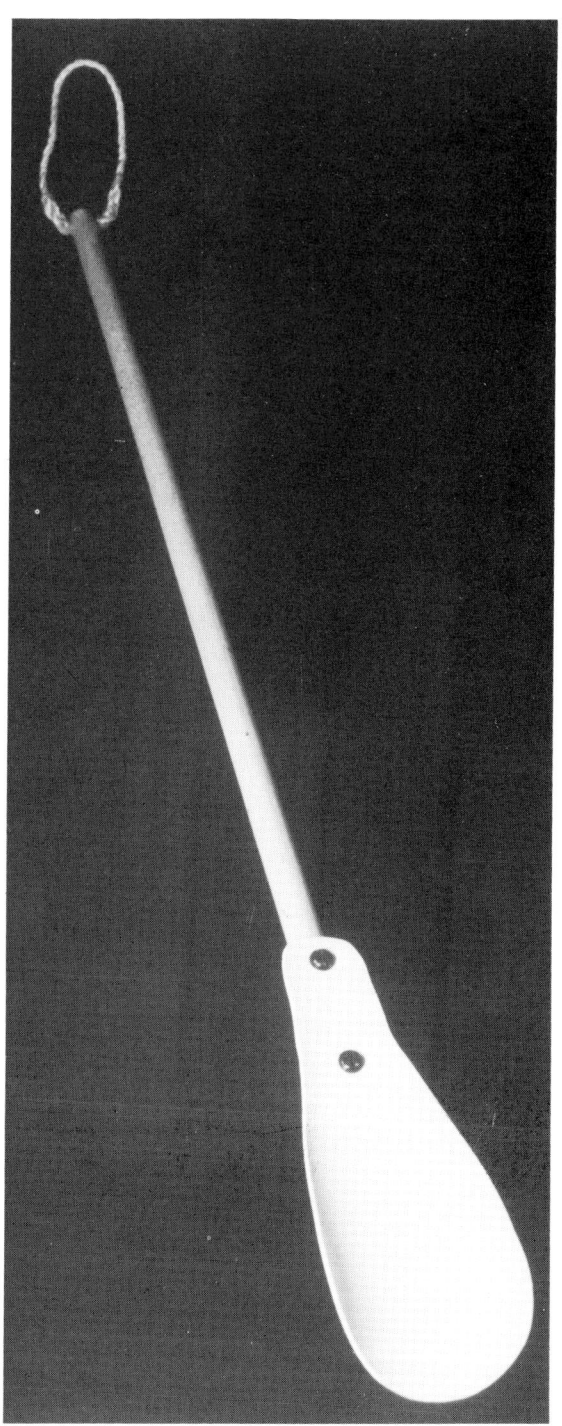

Plastic guttering and dowelling Extended Shoe Horn

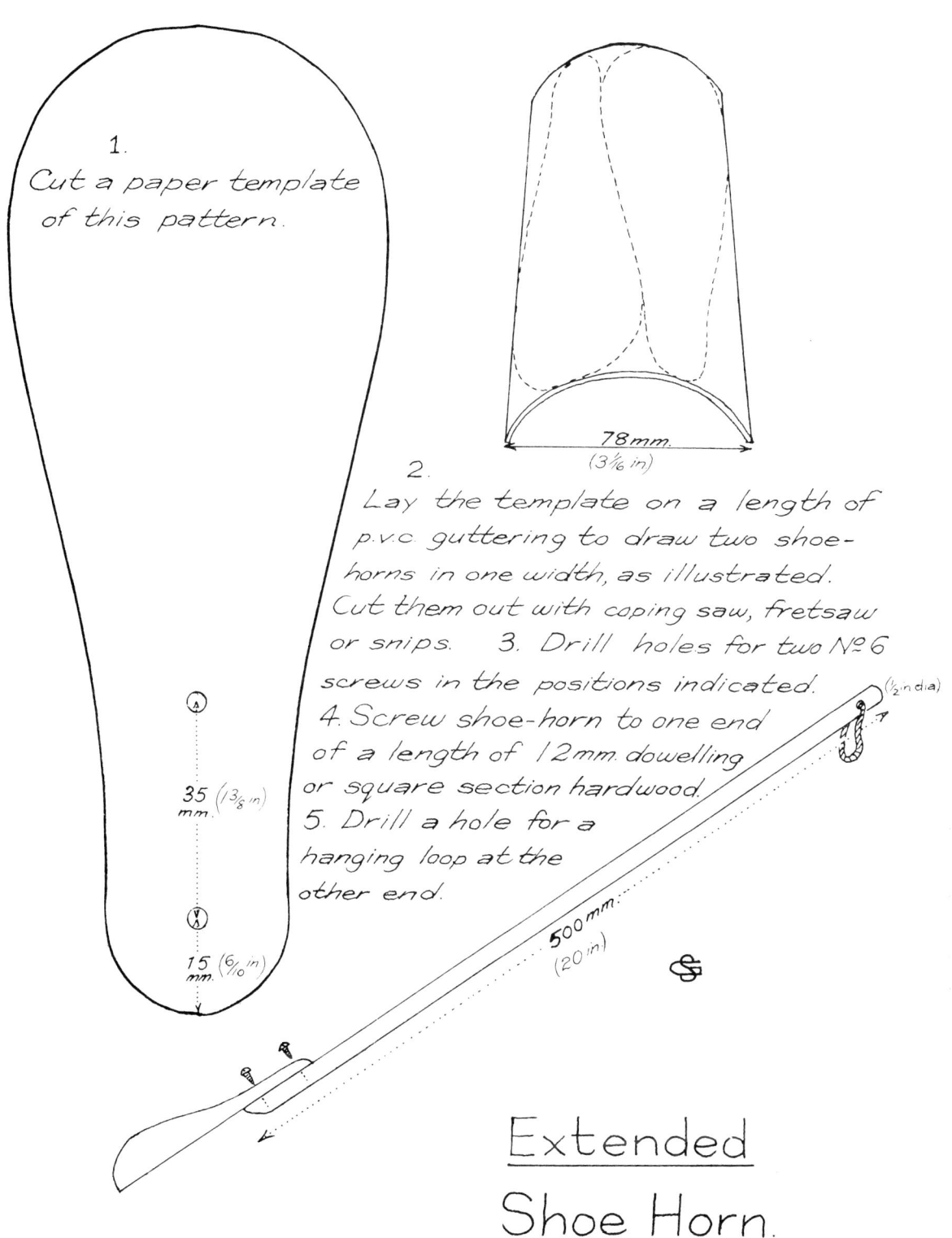

1.
Cut a paper template of this pattern.

78mm.
(3 ¹/₁₆ in)

2.
Lay the template on a length of p.v.c. guttering to draw two shoe-horns in one width, as illustrated. Cut them out with coping saw, fretsaw or snips. 3. Drill holes for two Nº 6 screws in the positions indicated. 4. Screw shoe-horn to one end of a length of 12mm. dowelling or square section hardwood. 5. Drill a hole for a hanging loop at the other end.

35 mm. (1³/₈ in)

15 mm. (⁶/₁₀ in)

(½ in dia)

500 mm.
(20 in)

Extended
Shoe Horn.

TIDY TROUGH

The blind and all whose sight is bad can benefit greatly from any means whereby small items required on a work bench, desk or dressing table, such as screws, tacks, paper clips and pins, can be kept in orderly compartments, easily identifiable by touch. The Tidy Trough is a simple and inexpensive means of providing that facility. It is also very useful to anyone having difficulty in manipulation, for the shape of the Trough makes it easy to pick up anything lying in it. In fact Tidy Troughs are aids to be valued by all, with or without disability, and are permanently in evidence on the author's desk and work bench.

Tidy Troughs can be made to suit individual needs, so only essential dimensions have been specified in the drawing, and even these must necessarily depend upon the type and size of the plastic guttering used. That used by the author is three inches wide, and is made and marketed by Marley Ltd, but several other types are available, in grey, black or white plastic.

The dividers, the design of which also provides stabilising legs, are cut out with a coping saw or fret-saw, from any material of a suitable thickness and rigidity. Plywood of about 4 mm ($\frac{3}{16}$ in.) thickness is ideal, but plastic, fibreboard, and even metal sheet could be used, for the dividers are small enough to utilise offcuts of many materials that may be readily available.

It is important only to ensure that the glue used is of a suitable type. Manufacturers of plastic guttering usually market a glue that is compatible with their own product, so this does not present a problem normally. However, if you have any difficulty in this respect there are several brands of glue widely available in hardware and handyman shops formulated specifically for glueing PVC and any of these should prove satisfactory. It is necessary to glue the dividers at each end of the trough, but the rest can be left unglued, and thus infinitely adjustable, if this is likely to be more convenient.

Plywood dividers may be smoothed with glass-paper and then painted or varnished to make, out of really very little, a handsome piece of equipment and a most acceptable gift. One further point worthy of note is that these Troughs are stackable, one on top of the other, which can be helpful in saving space, particularly in a workshop.

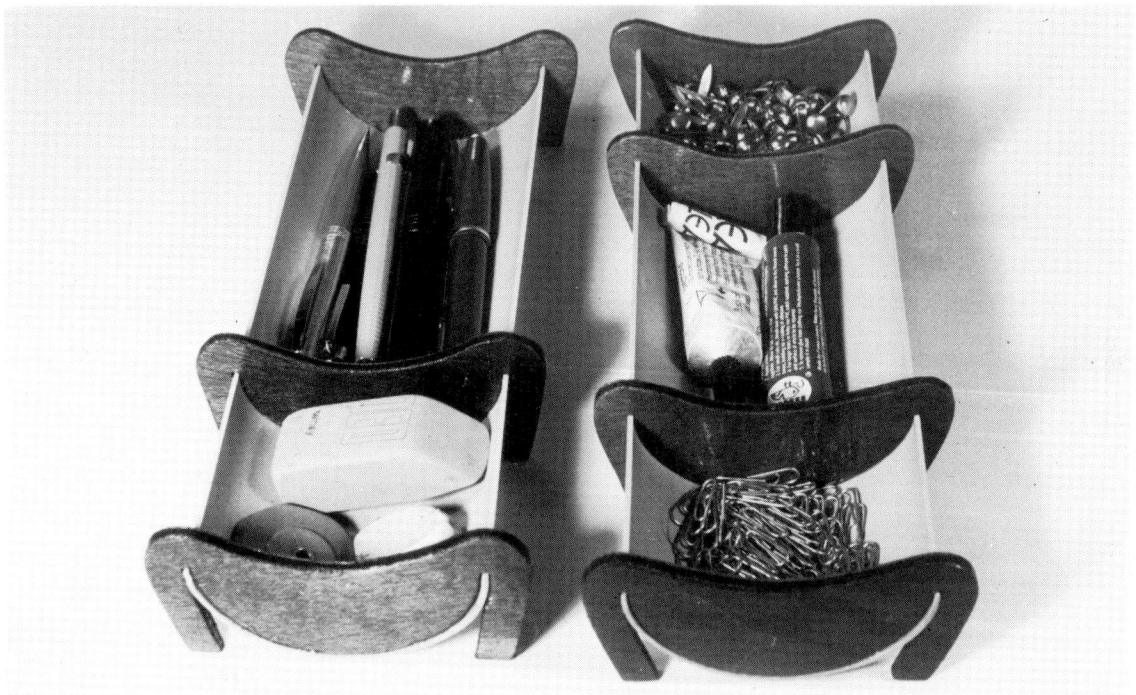

Tidy Troughs with typical contents

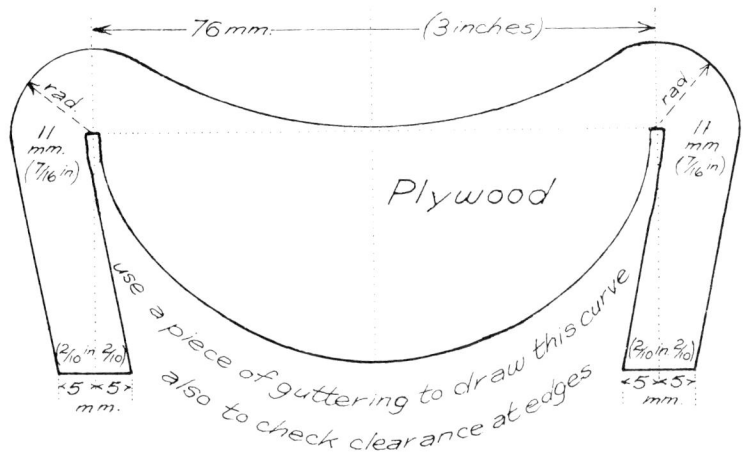

76 mm. (3 inches)

rad.

11 mm. (7/16 in)

Plywood

11 mm. (7/16 in)

use a piece of guttering to draw this curve
also to check clearance at edges

(2/10 in 2/10)

←5 × 5→ mm.

(2/10 in 2/10)

←5 × 5→ mm.

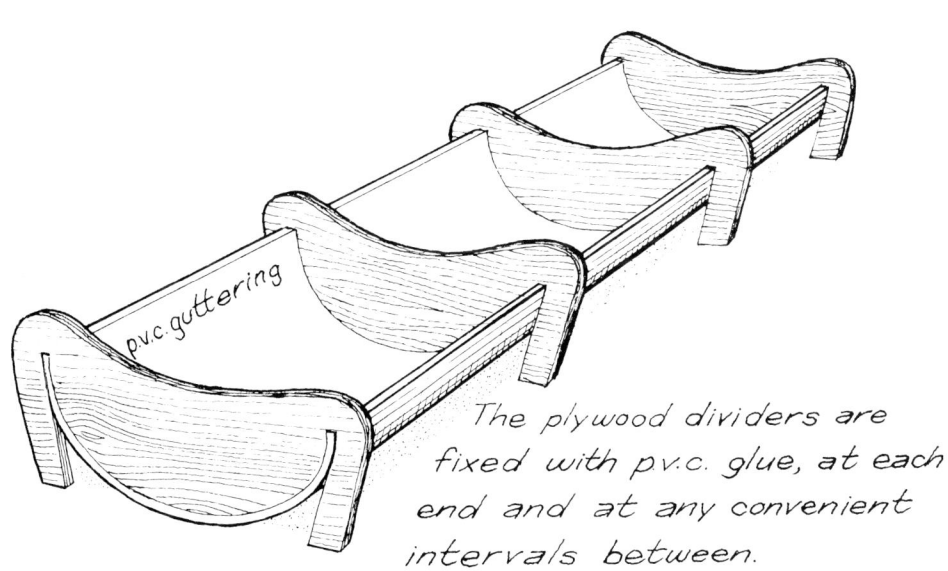

p.v.c. guttering

The plywood dividers are
fixed with p.v.c. glue, at each
end and at any convenient
intervals between.

Tidy Trough.

SOCK EASER

This very simple device is intended to help with the humdrum task of putting on socks or stockings, for there are a great many people who find it difficult to reach their toes. The open end of the sock or stocking is passed over the two parallel lengths of plastic guttering — Parts C in the diagram — which hold it open. The rest of the garment is then bunched up onto the guttering, until the toe is up to the lower end of the rectangular piece of plywood — Part A. Using the handle — Part B — the open end of the sock or stocking can now be placed over the foot, which slides downwards into the toe of the garment, and then the Easer can be slipped upwards and outwards over the heel leaving the garment in position on the foot. That completes what is generally regarded as the difficult procedure; the remainder of the operation, pulling the garment up the leg, is not usually a problem.

Components

Part A is a rectangle 140 x 50 mm ($5\frac{1}{2}$ x 2 in.) of 9 mm ($\frac{3}{8}$ in.) plywood, with the corners well rounded and the whole piece thoroughly sanded smooth. Four pilot holes for No. 8 screws are drilled as shown in the drawing.

Part B is a piece of 16 mm ($\frac{5}{8}$ in.) square section hardwood about 700 mm (28 in.) long, forming an extended handle. At the lower end a portion 120 x 4 mm ($4\frac{3}{4}$ in x $\frac{3}{16}$ in.) is cut away, and two countersunk holes are drilled through it 70 mm ($2\frac{3}{4}$ in.) apart. The lower end of the component is rounded off and the whole is thoroughly sanded smooth.

Parts C, of which two are required, are 80 mm ($3\frac{1}{8}$ in.) lengths of 78 mm ($3\frac{1}{16}$ in.) wide plastic guttering. Midway along the length of each, and about 14 mm ($\frac{9}{16}$ in.) in from the edge, a countersunk hole is drilled to accommodate a No. 8 screw. The corners are well rounded off and all rough edges sanded smooth.

NOTE: using only one screw for each Part C allows a degree of pivoting about the mid point, which some users find to be advantageous; however, if a user prefers complete rigidity, an extra screw through each Part C will easily accomplish this.

Assembly

Part A fits centrally into the cut away portion at the lower end of Part B and is fixed in position with two countersunk No. 8 x 16 or 19 mm ($\frac{5}{8}$ or $\frac{3}{4}$ in.) screws, passing through from the underside of Part B upwards into two of the pilot holes in Part A. The two Parts C are fixed into position on the top of Part A with two (or four if preferred — see Note above) No. 8 x 10 mm ($\frac{3}{8}$in.) countersunk screws passing through Parts C from above, downwards into two pilot holes in Part A.

Finishing

It is essential that all parts of this device are compIetly smooth to avoid snagging, but varnishing or painting the wood is not really necessary.

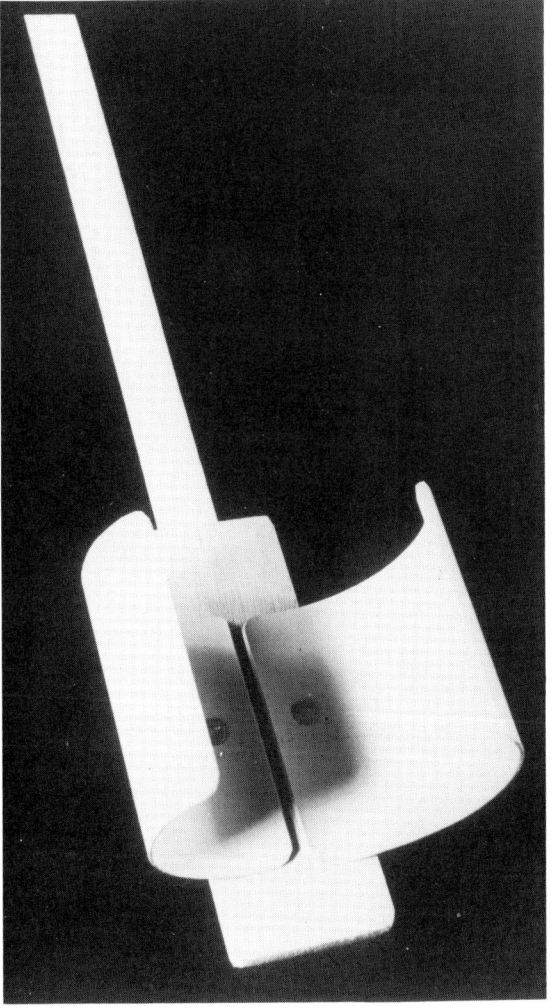

Sock Easer

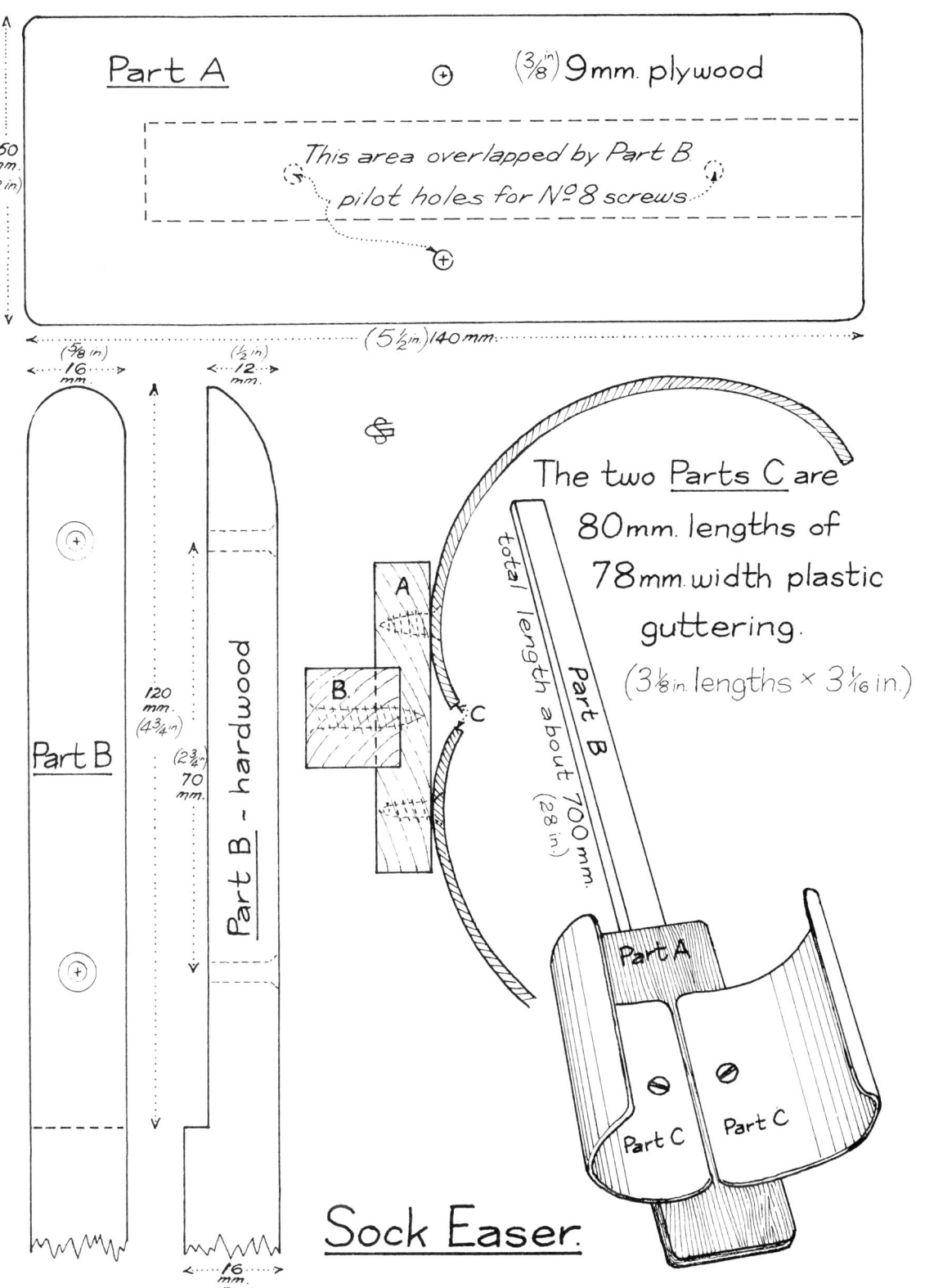

Part A   ⊕ $(\tfrac{3}{8}in)$ 9mm. plywood

50 mm. (2 in)

This area overlapped by Part B.
pilot holes for Nº 8 screws

$(5\tfrac{1}{2}in.)$ 140 mm.

$(\tfrac{5}{8}in)$ 16 mm.

$(\tfrac{1}{2}in)$ 12 mm.

Part B

Part B ~ hardwood

120 mm. $(4\tfrac{3}{4}in)$

$(2\tfrac{3}{4}")$ 70 mm.

A

B

C

total length about 700 mm. (28 in.)

Part B

The two Parts C are
80mm. lengths of
78mm. width plastic
guttering.
$(3\tfrac{1}{8}in.$ lengths × $3\tfrac{1}{16}in.)$

Part A

Part C   Part C

16 mm. $(\tfrac{5}{8}in)$

Sock Easer.

WRIST STRAPS FOR STICKS

Anyone who constantly has to use a stick knows the irritating necessity of 'parking' it, on the back of a chair or the edge of a table, in order to free temporarily the hand that was holding it, only to hear it clatter to the floor. This irritation can be avoided by providing a wrist strap near the top of the stick so that, when the hand is needed, the stick is readily suspended from the wrist, immediately retrievable.

There are several ways in which such a wrist strap may be attached to a stick. A short length of cord, leather strap, bootlace or tape can be bound to the top, as illustrated, by means of a seizing. An even simpler method is to bind it on with adhesive tape, but this tends to become sticky and messy after a while, so has to be replaced frequently. One method to be avoided is to use tacks, nails, drawing pins or staples, because any piercing of the stick at this critical point will inevitably weaken it, apart from permanently marking it.

A split spiral or a spring tool clip with a loop of cord or strap attached to it allows the strap to be attached to and removed from any stick without it being a permanent fixture, which is particularly useful for those who like to change their sticks for different occasions, as many stick users do. The Turk's Head Wrist Strap can also be slipped off one stick and onto another, or be removed for washing, without disturbing the construction of the knot.

Turk's Head wrist strap

For anyone who can master this knot — and the Turk's Head illustrated is the simplest of a very large family of knots — it provides a wrist strap of most elegant appearance and practical form. The knot

shown in the drawings is described as a three lead, four bight, tripled Turk's Head. Three lead, because the cord passes three times around the stick to complete the basic knot; four bight, because the cord passes from one side of the basic knot to the other four times during its construction; tripled, because the cord is led three times around the complete basic knot.

Cut a length of stout cord, between 3 mm ($\frac{1}{8}$ in.) and 5 mm ($\frac{3}{16}$ in.) in diameter and about 400 mm (16 in.) long. Seal the ends with strips of adhesive tape or glue so that they do not fray out whilst working. Lay the approximate centre of the cord across the stick and, carefully following 1, tie the first step, using the end indicated by the arrows. 2 shows the transposition of the two loops on the top of the stick, the left loop being lifted over the right loop. When this transposition has been completed, the knot appears as in (3), in which the arrows indicate the third step. (4) shows the completion of the basic knot, everything following being a comparatively simple matter of doubling and then trebling the original lead. The start of this process is shown in (5) and it consists of repeating the steps shown in (1), (2) & (3) a second time, remembering that the end with which you are working must always stay on the same side of the original lead. In the illustrations, the doubling process is shown placed to the left of the original line.

At the stage represented in (6) the doubling process is complete and the wrist loop is formed, using the other end of the line from that which was used hitherto. A loop, sufficiently large to pass a hand through, is left free, the remainder of the line being used to triple the Turk's Head, working in the

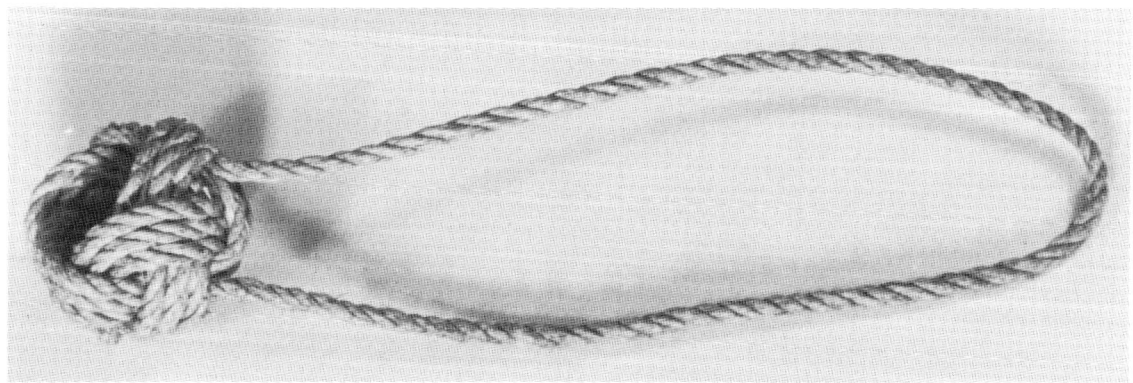

Turk's Head Wrist Strap removed from its stick

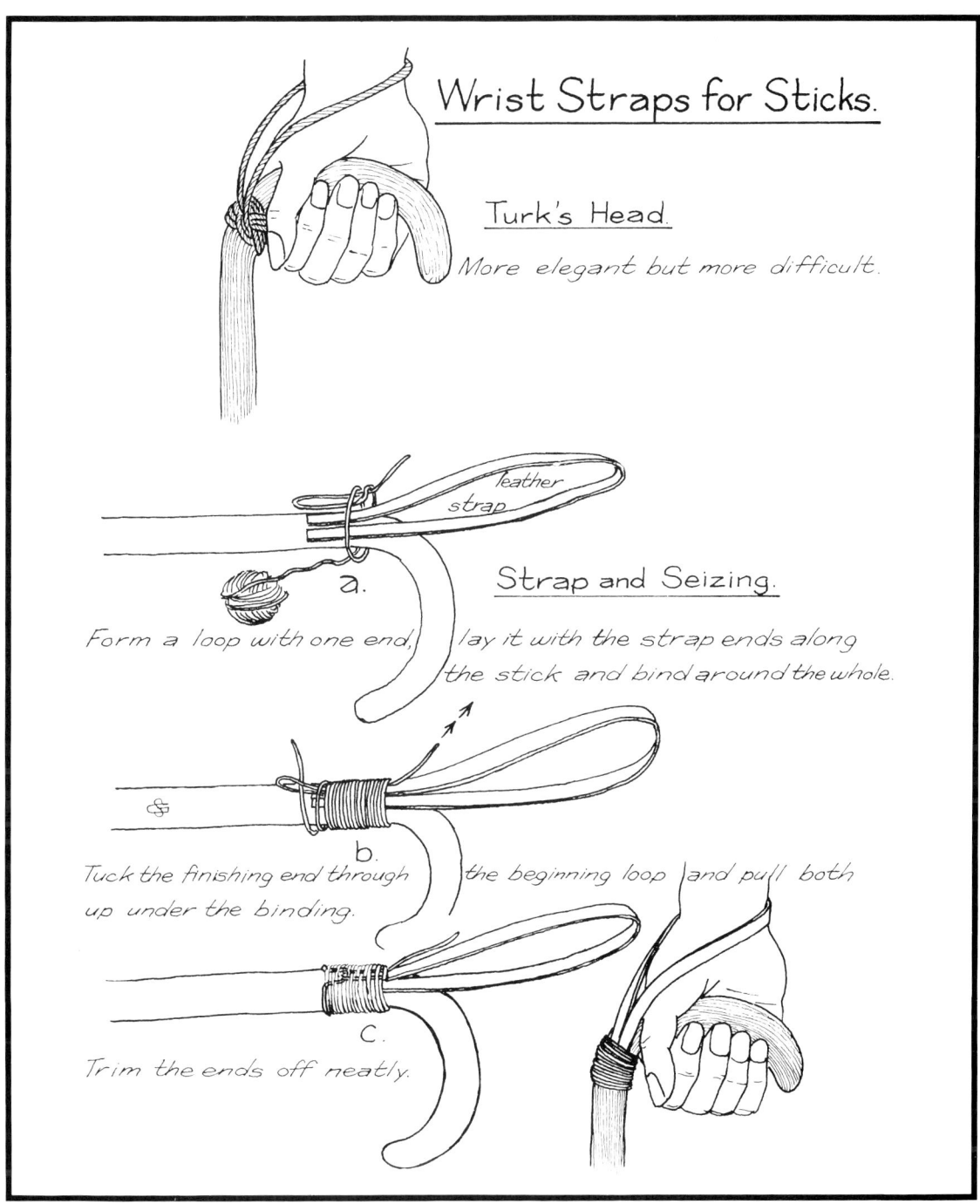

Wrist Straps for Sticks.

Turk's Head.

More elegant but more difficult.

Strap and Seizing.

a. *Form a loop with one end,* *lay it with the strap ends along the stick and bind around the whole.*

b. *Tuck the finishing end through up under the binding.* *the beginning loop and pull both*

c. *Trim the ends off neatly.*

opposite direction from that followed by the first end, and on the other side of the original lead. The knot has to be worked tight at this stage, and it will be found easier to do this using a pair of pliers, as shown in (7). When the knot has been tripled completely, and all looseness worked out to one end or the other, place a drop of glue to secure each end of the line. Cut the remainder off close against the knot. If this is done carefully, the ends should be virtually invisible. You are left with the wrist loop secured by the Turk's Head firmly around the stick, but it will be possible to slide the knot down and off the stick, if and when this is necessary, without spoiling its construction.

Turk's Head Wrist Strap for a Stick.

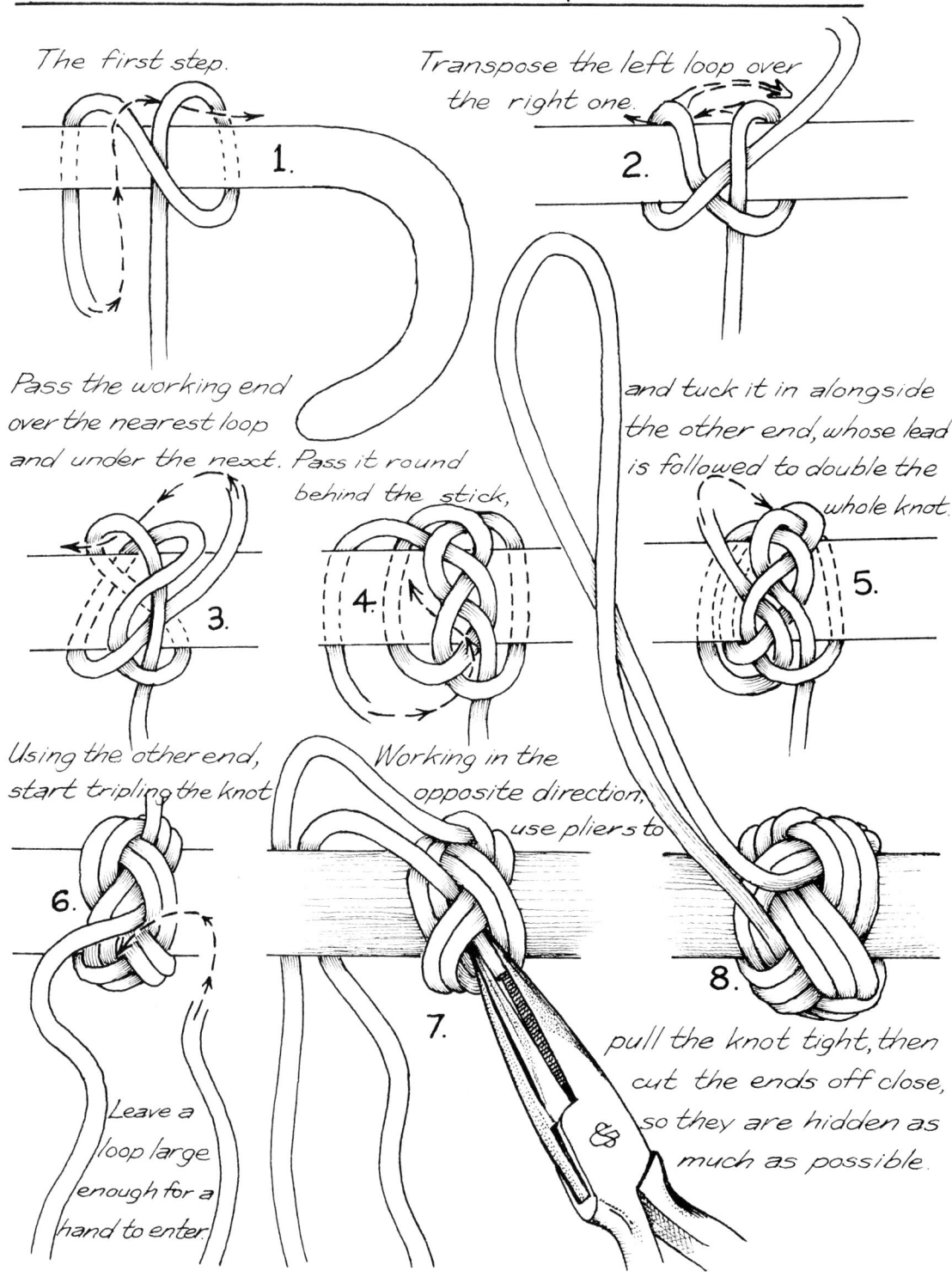

The first step.

1.

Transpose the left loop over the right one.

2.

Pass the working end over the nearest loop and under the next. Pass it round behind the stick,

3.

4.

and tuck it in alongside the other end, whose lead is followed to double the whole knot.

5.

Using the other end, start tripling the knot

6.

Leave a loop large enough for a hand to enter.

Working in the opposite direction, use pliers to

7.

8.

pull the knot tight, then cut the ends off close, so they are hidden as much as possible.

URINE BOTTLE RACK

Many gentlemen who are confined to wheelchairs are also obliged to use urine bottles. It can be very helpful for them to have a small supply of bottles stowed in a suitably positioned rack, in which clean and used bottles can be segregated. The Rack shown here can be made to provide as many spaces as may be required, by extending the horizontal length. The first two such Racks were produced for the Canal Street House Day Centre in Chester, England; each held up to ten bottles. For ordinary domestic purposes a four unit rack, as illustrated, seems about right.

Materials

The Bars for the Rack illustrated, which has two Vertical Bays to accommodate four bottles, are:
$(2 \times 110) + (2 \times 9) + 4$ mm = 242 mm in length, or
$(2 \times 4\frac{3}{8}) + (2 \times \frac{3}{8}) + \frac{5}{32}$ in. = $9\frac{21}{32}$ in.

The two Vertical Elements at each end of the Rack are cut from thicker plywood than the rest. For each Vertical Element allow 255 x 193 mm $(10\frac{1}{16} \times 7.6$ in.). The Ends should be cut from 9 mm $(\frac{3}{8}$ in.) plywood, the Dividers from 4 mm $(\frac{5}{32}$ in.) plywood.

The Horizontal Elements or Bars are equal lengths of 8 mm $(\frac{5}{16}$ in.) diameter hardwood dowelling. Allow to each Bar 110 mm $(4\frac{3}{8}$ in.) clearance per Vertical Bay plus the thickness of all the Vertical Elements.

Construction

Make a cardboard template, from which all the Vertical Elements can be marked out, including the positions in which the holes are to be drilled. All the necessary dimensions are provided in the drawing on page 46. Draw the front and back vertical lines first, 193 mm (7.6 in.) apart, then draw the line joining the centres of the two front holes 9 mm $(\frac{3}{8}$ in.) in from the front vertical line and mark the centres 157 mm $(6\frac{3}{16}$ in.) apart. Now the angles of the lines joining the centres of the remaining holes and radii can be plotted, using a protractor. The radii are then drawn and joined by straight lines where indicated.

Using this template, cut two Ends out of 9 mm $(\frac{3}{8}$ in.) plywood and drill the holes into their inner faces to a depth of about 6 mm $(\frac{1}{4}$ in.). Cut as many Dividers as are required and drill the holes right through them. Cut eight lengths of dowelling to the appropriate length, as indicated above, and glue them into place in the holes in one of the End Verticals. Slide the Dividing Vertical or Verticals onto the Horizontal Bars and then glue the free ends of the Bars into the other End Vertical. Ensure that the two Ends and the Bars are all square and allow the glue to set hard before attempting to position the Dividers accurately.

Once the Ends and Bars are set firmly, the position of the Divider or Dividers can be marked out on the Horizontal Bars, using a pencil and measuring rule to establish the clearance of 110 mm $(4\frac{3}{8}$ in.) between Verticals. Apply a little glue around each Bar in the position indicated and, when all eight Bars have been thus treated, slide the Divider into place and allow the glue to set hard.

Finishing

It is important that an Aid of this kind should be kept perfectly clean by regular washing. Therefore it must be sanded down smooth, sealed and then covered with at least three coats of paint or varnish before it is put into use. The Rack may be screwed to a wall using small wooden blocks as indicated in the sketch. Alternatively, and perhaps better, large cup hooks may be screwed into the wall and the Rack hung upon them by engaging the rear Horizontal Bars on the hooks. Fitted in this way, the Rack can be detached easily for washing.

The Horizontal Elements are all made of 8mm. (5/16 in.) diameter hardwood dowelling.

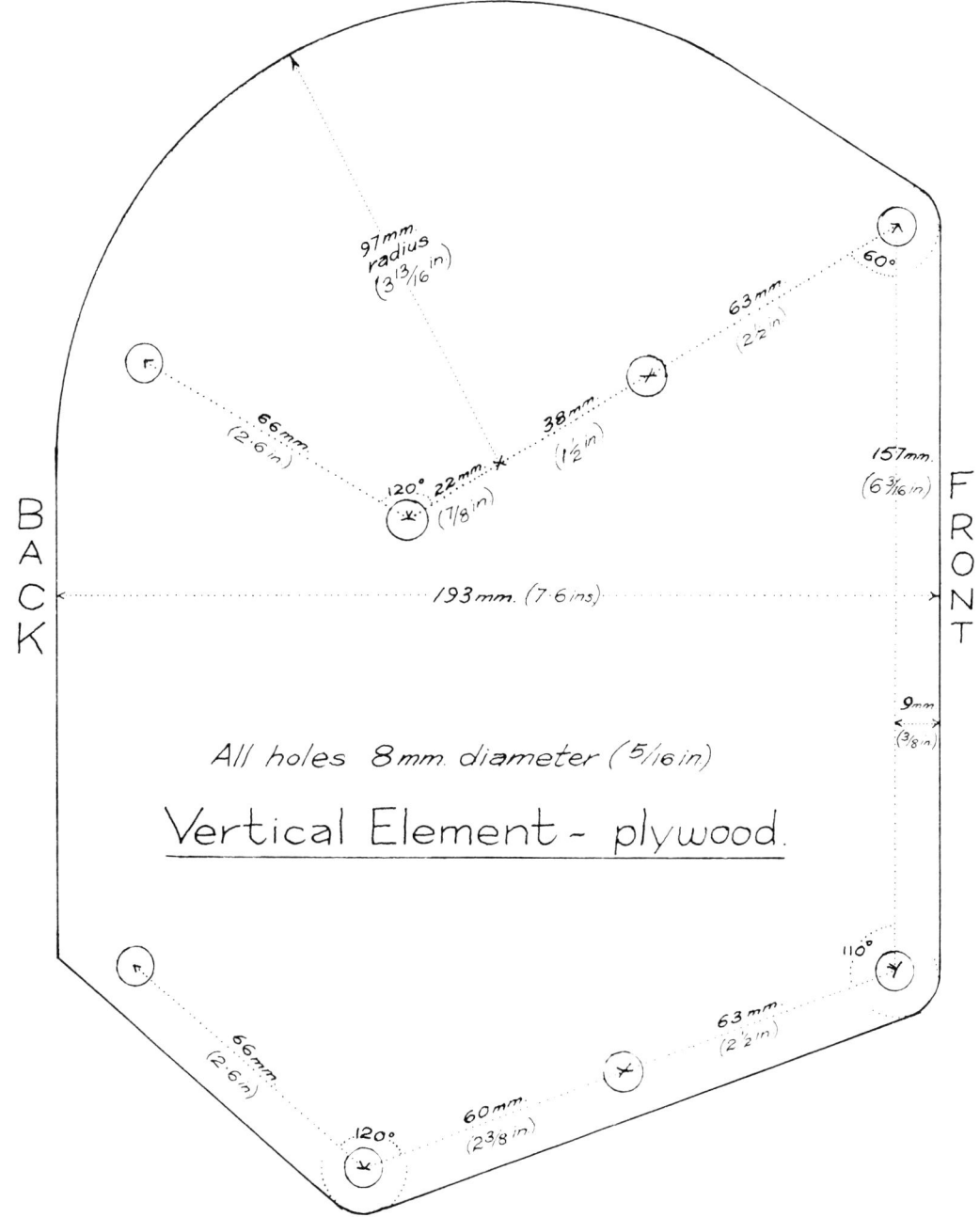

97mm. radius (3¹³/₁₆ in.)

63mm. (2½ in.)

66mm. (2.6 in)

38mm. (1½ in.)

120° 22mm. (⁷/₈ in.)

60°

157mm. (6³/₁₆ in.)

B A C K

F R O N T

193mm. (7.6 ins.)

9mm. (³/₈ in.)

All holes 8mm. diameter (⁵/₁₆ in.)

Vertical Element - plywood.

110°

66mm. (2.6 in)

63mm. (2½ in.)

120° 60mm. (2³/₈ in.)

Urine Bottle Rack.

Scale 2:3.

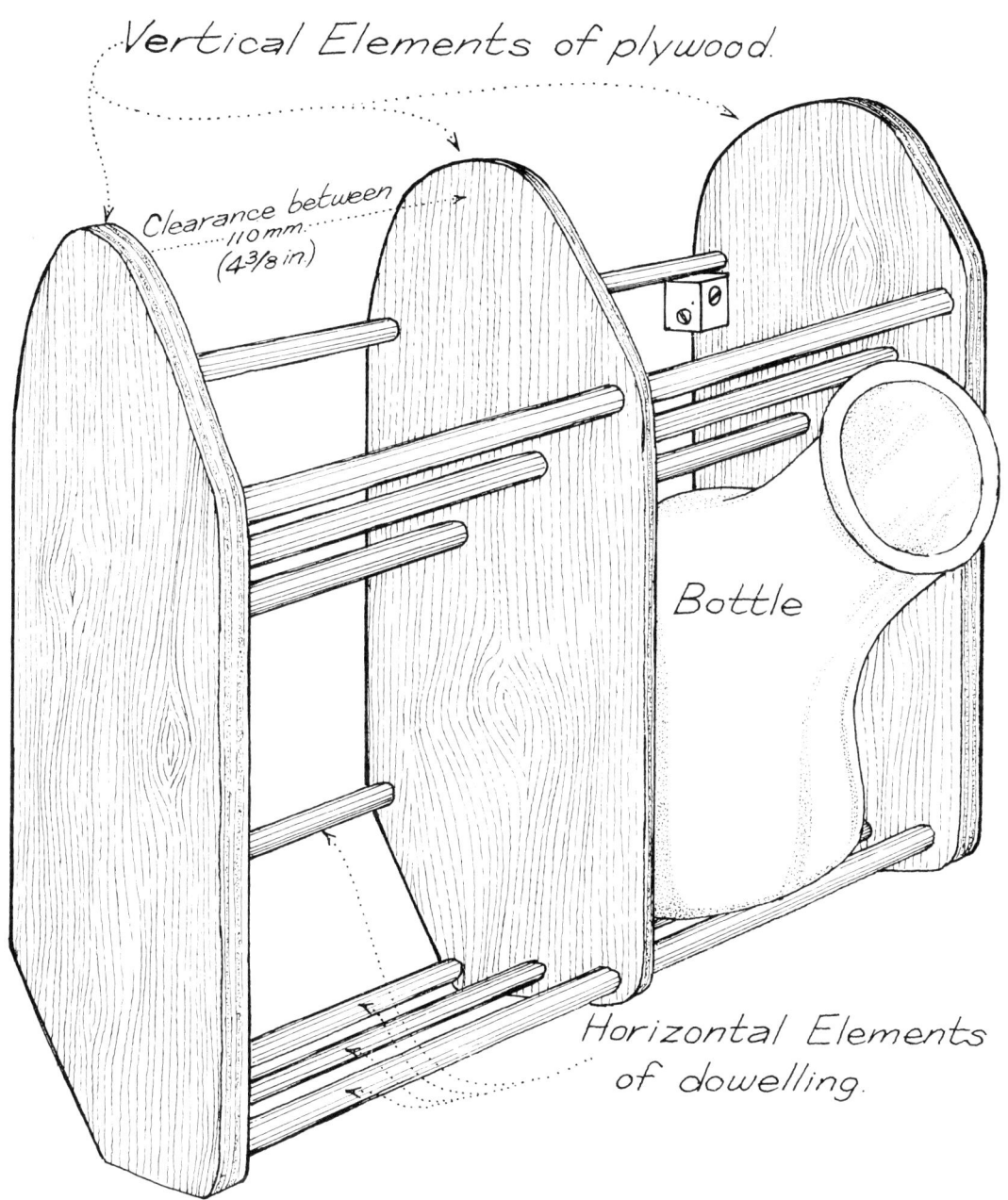

Vertical Elements of plywood.

Clearance between 110 mm. (4 3/8 in)

Bottle

Horizontal Elements of dowelling.

Urine Bottle Rack.

REACHER

The principal purpose of the Reacher is to provide a means whereby anyone confined to a wheelchair or bed can reach out and pick up small, fiddly items that may have been dropped by accident, or have been placed beyond normal reach. A number of such devices are commercially manufactured and available from retailers and social services; however, those known to the author, whilst good for general purposes, lack the delicacy of touch which is required to pick up a dropped pin or needle, for instance, and smooth, slippery items, such as a plastic knitting needle or ballpoint pen, which can also present problems. The design offered here is, despite first appearances, very simple to make and to use, and provides great delicacy of movement.

Unlike most commercially available items, it is also inexpensive.

Components and materials

The necessary components are:

Part A 3 Claws — (Plastic sheet about 2 mm ($\frac{3}{32}$ in.) thick).

Part B 3 Claw Arms — (About 200 mm (8 in.) of angle section).

Part C 1 Junction Block — (80 x 70 x 20 mm (3 x $2\frac{3}{4}$ x $\frac{3}{4}$ in.)

Part D 1 Washer — (Plastic, metal or plywood).

Part E 1 Piston — (6 mm ($\frac{1}{4}$ in.) plywood about 50 mm (2 in.) square).

Reacher Components.

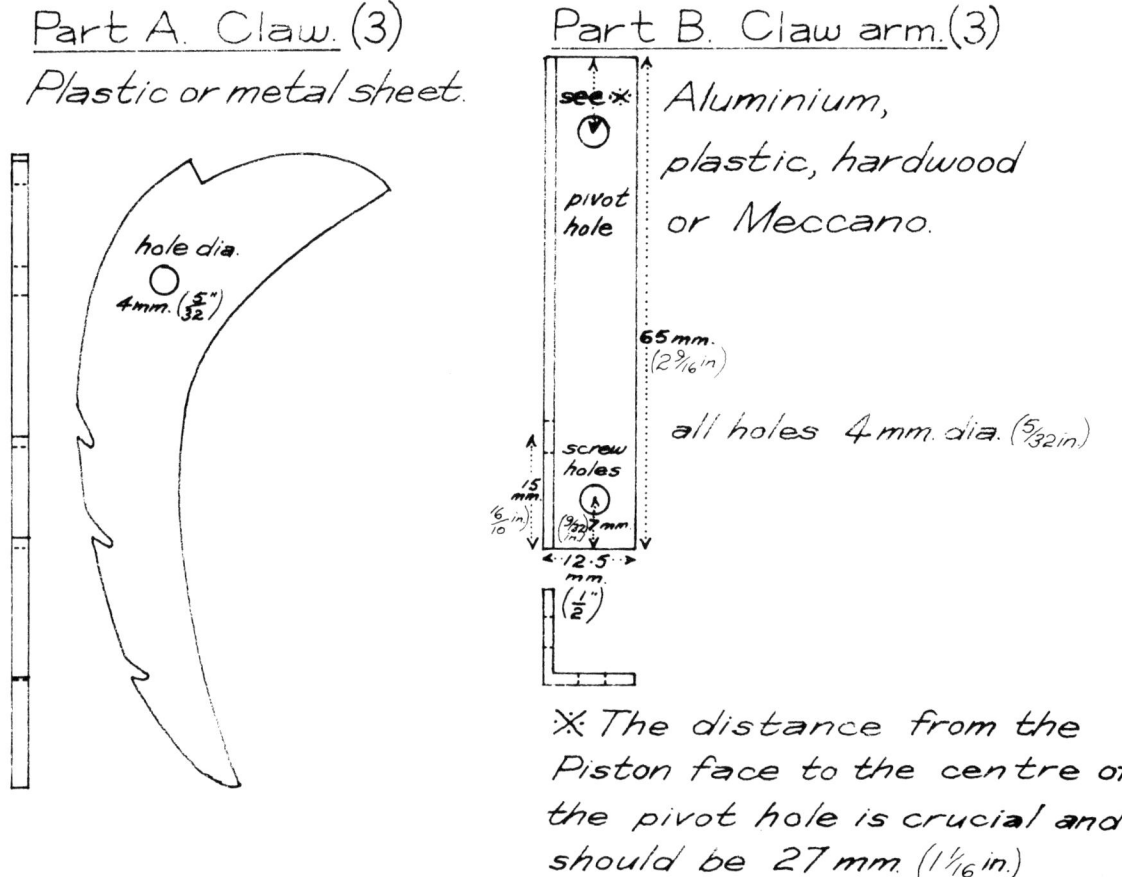

Part A. Claw. (3)
Plastic or metal sheet.

hole dia.
4 mm. ($\frac{5}{32}$")

Part B. Claw arm. (3)
see ✻
pivot hole

Aluminium, plastic, hardwood or Meccano.

65 mm. ($2\frac{9}{16}$ in)

all holes 4 mm. dia. ($\frac{5}{32}$ in)

screw holes

15 mm ($\frac{6}{10}$ in).

7 mm ($\frac{9}{32}$ in.)

12.5 mm ($\frac{1}{2}$")

✻ *The distance from the Piston face to the centre of the pivot hole is crucial and should be 27 mm. ($1\frac{1}{16}$ in.)*

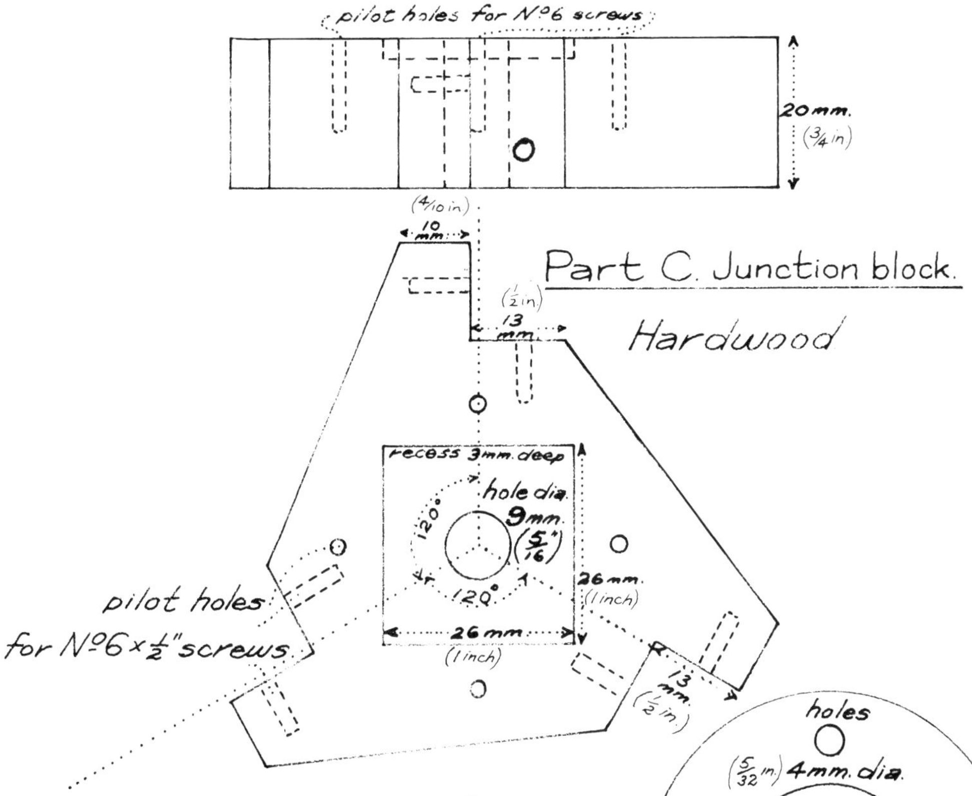

pilot holes for N°6 screws

20 mm. (¾ in)

(4/10 in)

10 mm

Part C. Junction block.

Hardwood

(½ in)

13 mm

recess 3mm deep

hole dia. 9mm ($\frac{5}{16}$")

120°

120°

26 mm (1 inch)

26 mm (1 inch)

13 mm (½ in)

pilot holes for N°6 × ½" screws

All parts drawn full size.

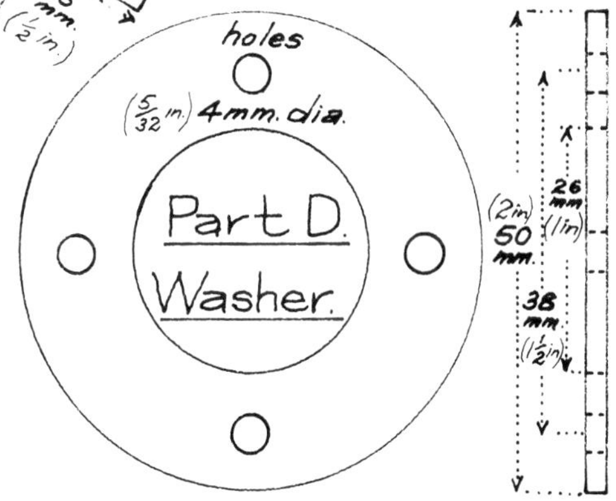

holes ($\frac{5}{32}$ in) 4mm. dia.

Part D. Washer.

(2in) 50 mm. — 26 mm (1in) — 38 mm (1½ in)

Plastic or metal sheet. (same material as Part A.)

Part F   1 Grip — (Plastic, metal or plywood sheet).
1 standard Hozelock patent garden hose connector.
Dowelling, 720 × 8 mm (28½ × $\frac{5}{16}$ in.) diameter.
Standard garden hose, 640 mm (25¼ in.) long.
10 No. 6 × 12 mm (½ in.) round head screws.
3 standard Meccano brass nuts and bolts (Parts Nos. 37b & c).
Elastic bands about 28 mm (1⅛ in.) long.

Parts A, D and F can be made from the same material, for example PVC, polypropylene, acrylic or other plastic sheet about 2 mm (⅛ in.) thick, cut to shape with a coping saw or fretsaw. Metal sheet, particularly aluminium, would be satisfactory also, but more difficult to cut. Thin plywood provides another alternative, but, if used for the claws — Part A — longer pivot bolts than the Meccano type specified would be needed.

Parts B — The Claw Arms   can be made from several materials also, but aluminium angle or Meccano angle provide the best choice, with plastic or hardwood angle as reasonable alternatives.

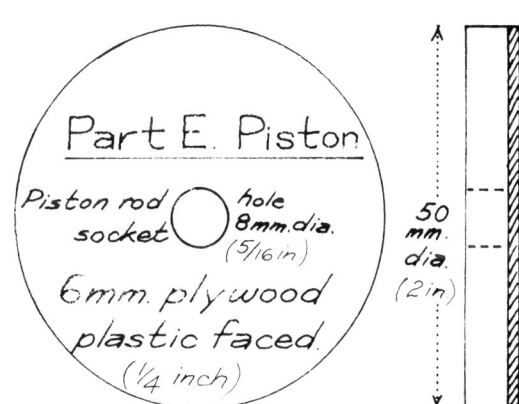

Part E. Piston

Piston rod socket

hole 8mm.dia. (5/16 in)

6mm. plywood plastic faced (¼ inch)

50 mm dia. (2 in)

Several kinds of aluminium, plastic and hardwood angle sections are sold in handyman shops, usually in 2 metre (6 ft) lengths, but it is often sold in shorter lengths as well for use as picture framing. The angle should be about 12 mm ($\frac{1}{2}$ in.) wide on each leg.

Part C -- the Junction Block should be of hardwood, about 20 mm ($\frac{3}{4}$ in.) thick. Transfer the plan by tracing from the drawing and cut carefully with a tenon saw or jigsaw. Drill the central hole. Remove the square recess with a chisel.

Part E -- the Piston is a disc of 6 mm ($\frac{1}{4}$ in.) plywood or similar material, cut with a coping saw or fretsaw, and it has a central 8 mm ($\frac{5}{16}$ in.) diameter hole, into which the length of dowelling, which acts as the piston rod, fits flush. To reduce friction in operation it is worthwhile facing the piston with a suitable plastic material, cut to the same diameter and glued in place.

The Hose which forms the outer sleeve, is ordinary plastic garden hose, widely available in hardware, gardening and handyman shops. An old leaky piece, no longer of use in the garden will do just as well as a new piece for this purpose.

The Hozelock Connector is as widely available as garden hose, from the same sources of supply. Only one connector is required, and it is carefully sawn into two halves across its centre section.

NOTE: providing that strength and rigidity of the materials used are adequate, the thickness is not important, so long as the drawn *plans* are followed accurately. If the Claws, Part A, are cut correctly, only one dimension is crucially important, namely the 27 mm ($1\frac{1}{16}$ in.) distance between the Piston face and the centres of the Claw Arm pivot holes. To ensure that these holes are correctly positioned, first screw the Claw Arms, Parts B, in the notches provided for them in Part C, the Junction Block. Place the Piston flat on the Junction Block, centrally between the three Claw Arms, and measure 27 mm ($1\frac{1}{16}$ in.) up each Arm from the face of the Piston, to mark the correct drilling position for each pivot hole. If these holes are not accurately placed, the Claws will not operate correctly.

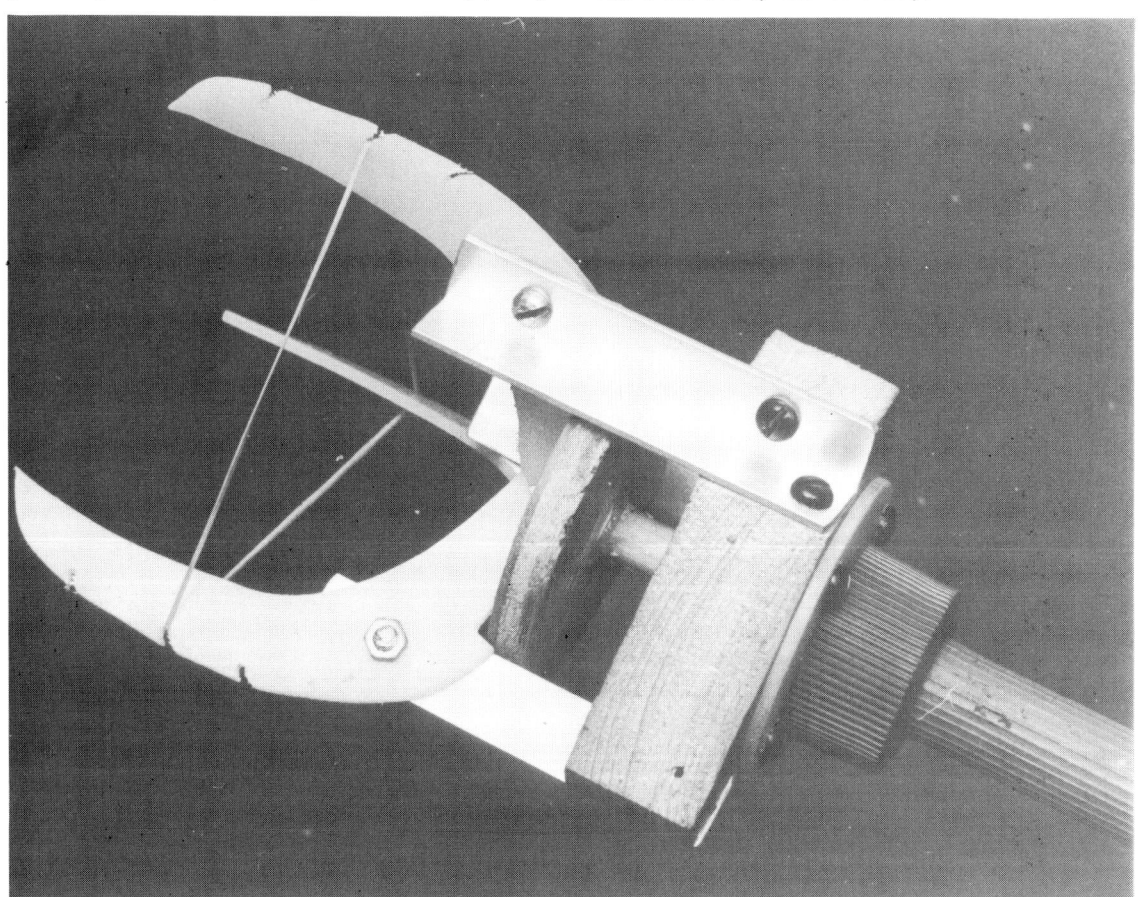

The Reacher's claw assembly

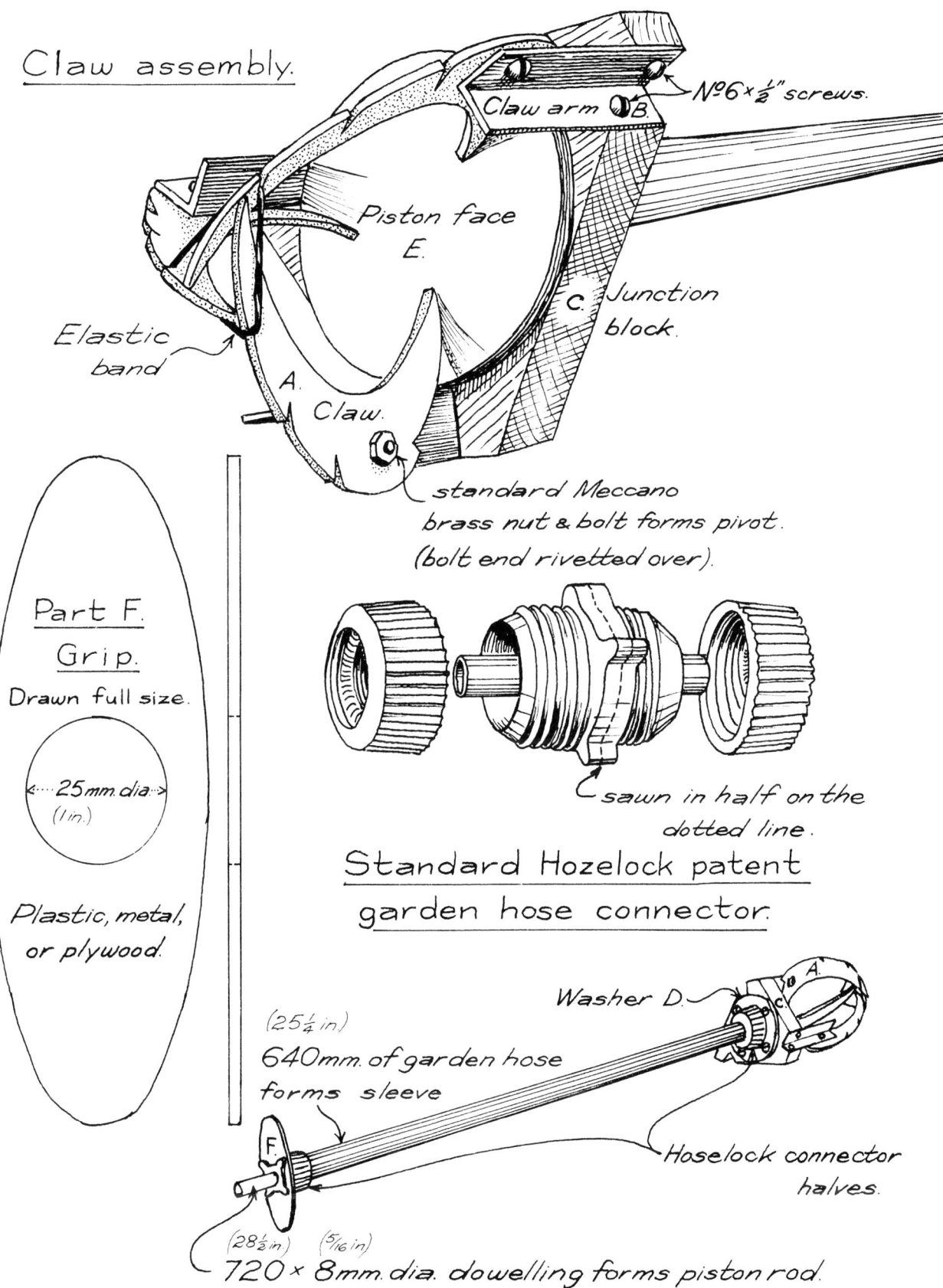

Claw assembly.

Nº6 × ½" screws.

Claw arm B.

Piston face E.

C. Junction block.

Elastic band

A. Claw.

standard Meccano
brass nut & bolt forms pivot.
(bolt end rivetted over).

Part F.
Grip.
Drawn full size.

25mm. dia.
(1 in.)

Plastic, metal,
or plywood.

sawn in half on the
dotted line.

Standard Hozelock patent
garden hose connector.

Washer D.

A.

(25¼ in.)
640mm. of garden hose
forms sleeve

Hoselock connector
halves.

(28½ in.) (5⁄16 in.)
720 × 8mm. dia. dowelling forms piston rod.

Reacher Assembly.

Assembly

Having completed the procedure described under the above NOTE, continue as follows:

1 Bolt the Claws to the Claw Arms with a Meccano bolt through each pivot hole. Ensure that they swing freely, then rivet over the end of each bolt with a small ball pein hammer, to prevent the nut working loose.

2 Place the cut end of one half of the Hozelock Connector into the square recess in the Junction Block; remove the ribbed cap from the half Connector and place the Washer, Part D, over the threaded male section. Screw the Washer to the Junction Block with four No. 6 x 12 mm ($\frac{1}{2}$ in.) screws, thus securing the male half Connector.

3 Pass one end of the length of Hose through the Connector cap, and into the half Connector on the Junction Block. Replace the cap onto the thread and screw it up tightly, thus securing that end of the length of Hose.

4 Remove the cap from the other half Connector, place the central hole of the Grip, Part F, over the threaded male section, pass the free end of the Hose through the cap and into the half Connector, replace the cap and screw it up tightly, thus securing the Grip to the Hose.

5 Holding the Junction Block uppermost, with the Claws opened outwards, place the Piston into position beneath the Claws. Fold the Claws together above the Piston and fit the elastic band over the three Claws, so that it lies in the same notch of each Claw and holds them together.

6 Pass the length of 8 mm ($\frac{5}{16}$ in.) dowelling through the Grip, into the Hose and along it, through the Junction Block and enter its lower end into the socket hole in the Piston. Pressing the end of the dowelling which still projects above the Grip should now cause the Piston to open the Claws, which should spring open and then close again when pressure is released. When all operates satisfactorily, glue the dowelling into its socket in the Piston.

Using the Reacher

Some users will find it helpful to have a pressure bar or button fitted at the handle end of the piston rod. This is easily made from a piece of dowelling, square or half round section hardwood, about 20 mm ($\frac{3}{4}$ in.) wide and deep and about 80 mm ($3\frac{1}{8}$ in.) long, with an 8 mm ($\frac{5}{16}$ in.) hole or socket drilled centrally, into which the dowelling piston rod can be securely glued.

There are three notches in the back of each Claw, into which the elastic band can be positioned. This allows for objects of various sizes to be grasped. With the elastic band placed in the notches nearest to the points, an object as small as a needle can be picked up. Smooth round or cylindrical objects can also be held without slipping, because the elastic band and the Claws together encircle them completely. For multi-purpose use it may be found convenient to place the elastic band in the lowest notch of one claw and in intermediate notches of the other two claws. The Reacher will not hold objects heavier than about 280 grams (10 ounces), unless the strength of the elastic band is increased. This can be done by adding more elastic bands in all of the notches, when commensurately greater pressure is required to open the Claws.

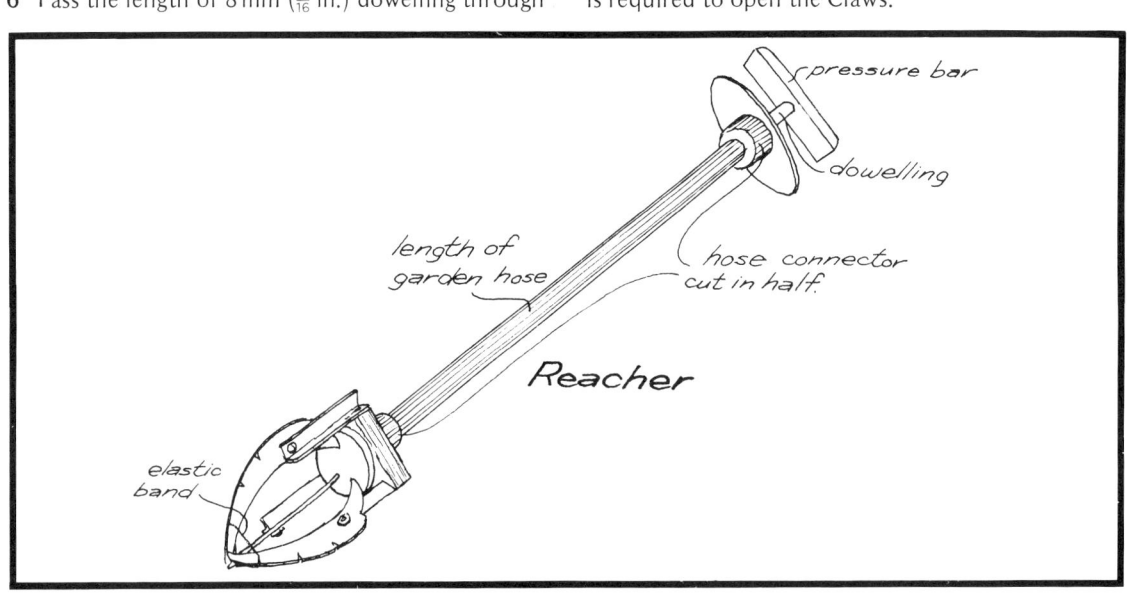

PIVOTING VICE

This is a particularly useful, yet inexpensive, aid for anyone with limited or no use of one arm. It can be clamped to the leg of virtually any kind of chair, including a wheel chair, and will hold an embroidery frame, small desk, easel, or other object to be worked upon. The jaws can be opened or closed, tilted from vertical to horizontal and pivoted through a full circle, with numerous intermediate positions, so this device's adaptability is considerable.

Although it sounds complicated it is in fact very simple, consisting of a few pieces of plywood, a length of standard square section hardwood, 80 cm ($31\frac{1}{2}$ in.) of standard polypropylene water pipe and a handful of screws and bolts.

Materials

80 cm ($31\frac{1}{2}$ in.) of polypropylene water pipe approximately 37 mm ($1\frac{1}{2}$ in.) outside diameter.

65 cm ($25\frac{5}{8}$ in.) of approximately 21 x 21 mm ($\frac{13}{16}$ in.) square section hardwood.

One piece of 9 mm ($\frac{3}{8}$ in.) plywood 150 x 114 mm (6 x $4\frac{1}{2}$ in.).

One piece of 9 mm ($\frac{3}{8}$ in.) plywood 250 x 21 mm ($9\frac{7}{8}$ x $\frac{13}{16}$ in.).

One piece of 6 mm ($\frac{1}{4}$ in.) plywood 120 x 100 mm ($4\frac{3}{4}$ x 4 in.).

3 screws No. 8 csk. x 20 to 25 mm ($\frac{3}{4}$ to $\frac{7}{8}$ in.).

2 screws No. 4 csk. x 12 to 15 mm ($\frac{1}{2}$ to $\frac{5}{8}$ in.).

2 bolts 6 x 65 mm ($\frac{1}{4}$ x $2\frac{1}{2}$ in.) with wing nuts and washers.

4 bolts 6 x 52 mm ($\frac{1}{4}$ x 2 in.) with wing nuts.

1 bolt 6 x 38 mm ($\frac{1}{4}$ x $1\frac{1}{2}$ in.) with nut and lock washer.

1 length of rod 6 mm x about 40 mm ($\frac{1}{4}$ x $1\frac{1}{2}$ in.) or an extra 38 mm ($1\frac{1}{2}$ in.) bolt.

About 200 mm (8 in.) thin cord or string.

1 Bulldog paper clip or sprung clothes peg.

Components and assembly

Part A – Socket Tube Make from 740 mm (29 in.) of polypropylene tube approximately 32 mm ($1\frac{1}{4}$ in.) inside diameter and approximately 37 mm ($1\frac{7}{16}$ in.) outside diameter. The tube used by the author is readily available in retail handyman shops,

and is stamped: 'Marley Extrusions 36 High Temp. PP. BS 5255', but any approximately similar tube will do equally well as the diameter is not critical. The top of the Socket Tube is slotted at intervals, as shown in the drawing, providing eight positions into which the pivoting head of the device can be locked.

Parts B1 and B2 – Locating Rings The purpose of these rings is to position the pivoting upright inside the socket tube so that it remains free to pivot and yet will not wobble or shake when the device is in use. The Locating Rings are two 30 mm ($1\frac{3}{16}$ in.) lengths of the same tube as is used for Part A. About 12 mm ($\frac{1}{2}$ in.) is cut out of the circumference of both rings, so that they can be compressed and fit snugly inside Part A. A hole, countersunk on the outside, is drilled through the mid point of each ring opposite to the cut-away section; into these holes screws are placed to hold the Locating Rings onto Part C, the Pivoting Upright.

Part C – Pivoting Upright Made from a 300 mm (1 ft) length of standard square section hardwood, approximately 21 mm x 21 mm ($\frac{13}{16}$ in. x $\frac{13}{16}$ in.). Pilot holes are drilled into the same face at 15 mm ($\frac{3}{5}$ in.) and 105 mm ($4\frac{1}{8}$ in.) from one end – which will be the lower end – to accept the No. 4 x 12 mm ($\frac{1}{2}$ in.) countersunk head screws, with which the Locating Rings – Parts B1 and B2 – are attached. In order that the Locating Rings will compress satisfactorily, the corners of the square section hardwood in the way of the Locating Rings must be pared away with a rasp or plane to produce an octagonal section through the Rings. A No. 8 round head brass screw is placed about 35 mm ($1\frac{3}{8}$ in.) above the upper locating ring screw and in a face at right angles to the locating ring screws; the head of this round head screw is left about 10 mm ($\frac{3}{8}$ in.) clear of the wood surface. When assembled the Pivoting Upright slides down inside the Socket Tube, with the Locating Rings compressed, and the protruding No. 8 screw drops into one of the slots cut into the top of the Socket Tube, thus acting as a pivot lock.

Part D – Upper Jaw of Vice Made from a 350 mm ($13\frac{3}{4}$ in.) length of 21 mm ($\frac{13}{16}$ in.) square section hardwood, this Part forms the vertical pivoting arm, as well as the upper jaw of the vice. It is tapered at one end and rounded at the other, both shapes in the same plane, the rounded end being the captive end of the pivot. Holes are drilled through the arm,

Pivoting Vice - clamps to chair leg.

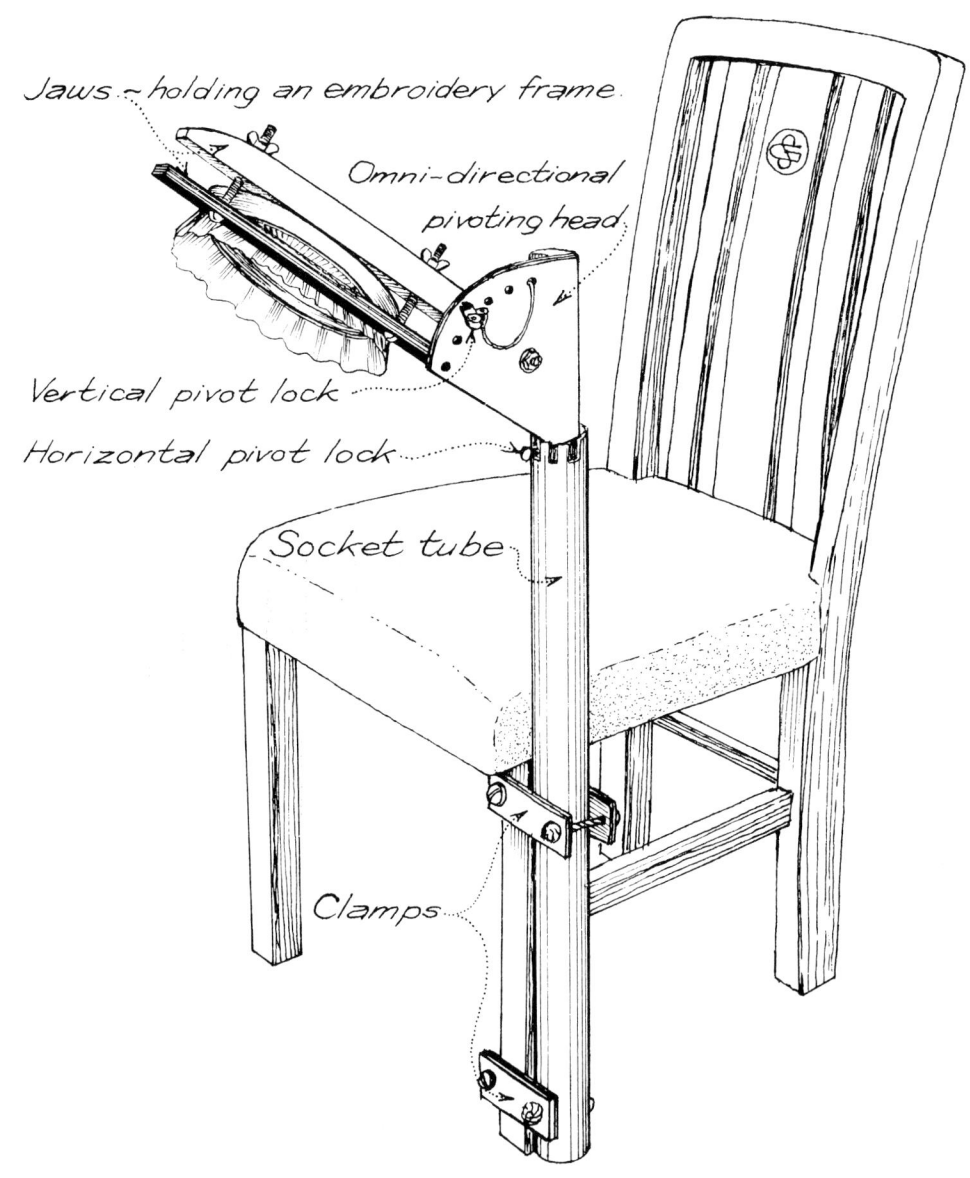

Jaws ~ holding an embroidery frame.

Omni-directional
pivoting head.

Vertical pivot lock

Horizontal pivot lock

Socket tube

Clamps

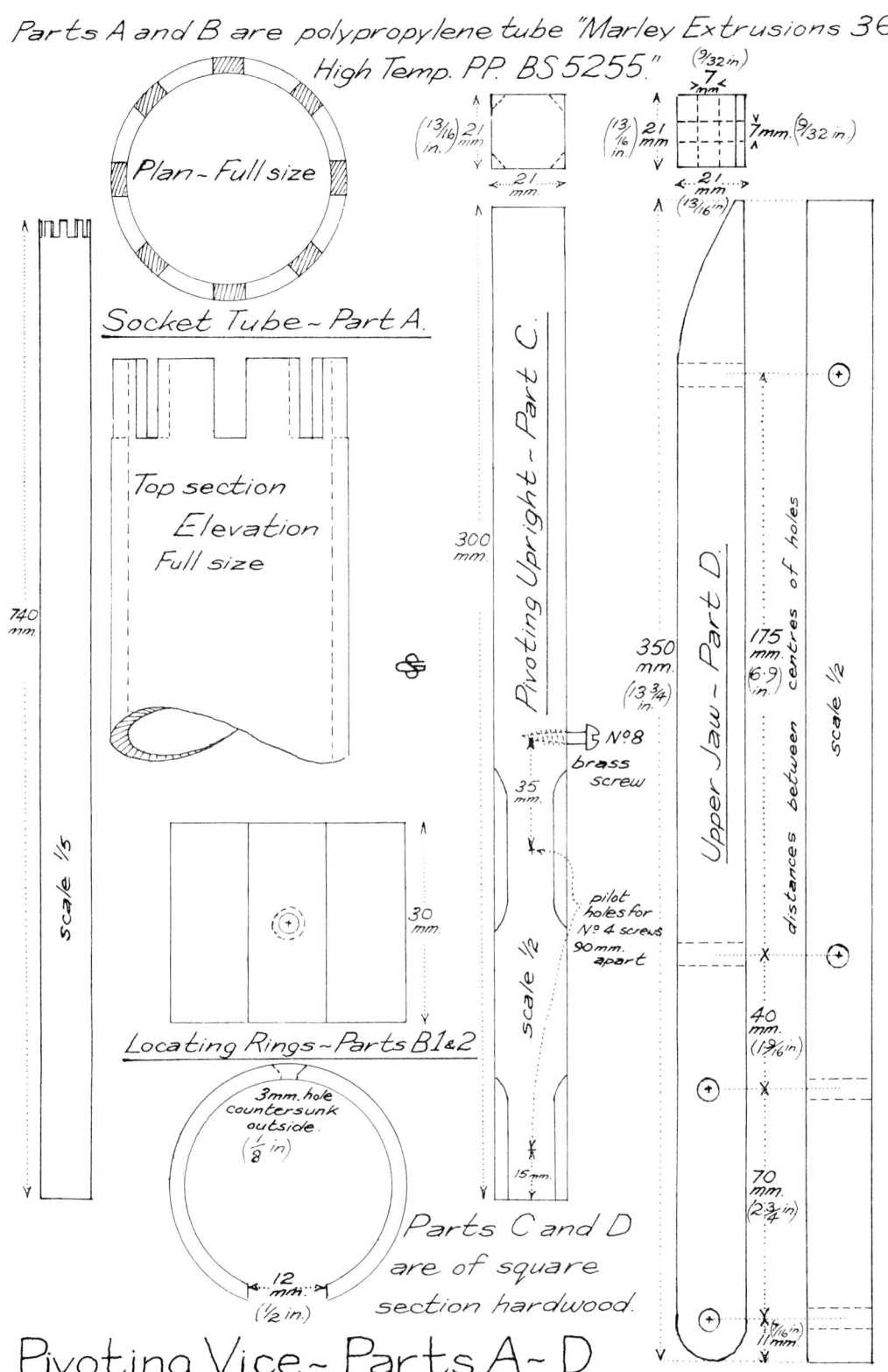

Parts A and B are polypropylene tube "Marley Extrusions 36 High Temp. P.P. BS 5255."

Plan ~ Full size

Socket Tube ~ Part A.

Top section

Elevation

Full size

740 mm

scale ⅕

Locating Rings ~ Parts B1 & 2

30 mm.

3mm. hole countersunk outside. (⅛ in)

12 mm (½ in.)

Pivoting Upright ~ Part C.

300 mm

350 mm (13¾ in.)

35 mm.

Nº8 brass screw

pilot holes for Nº 4 screws 90 mm. apart

scale ½

15 mm

(13/16 in.) 21 mm

21 mm

(13/16 in.) 21 mm

21 mm

(9/32 in.) 7 mm

7 mm (9/32 in.)

21 mm (13/16 in.)

Upper Jaw ~ Part D.

distances between centres of holes

175 mm (6.9 in.)

scale ½

40 mm (1 9/16 in.)

70 mm (2¾ in.)

7/16 in. 11 mm

Parts C and D are of square section hardwood.

Pivoting Vice ~ Parts A ~ D.

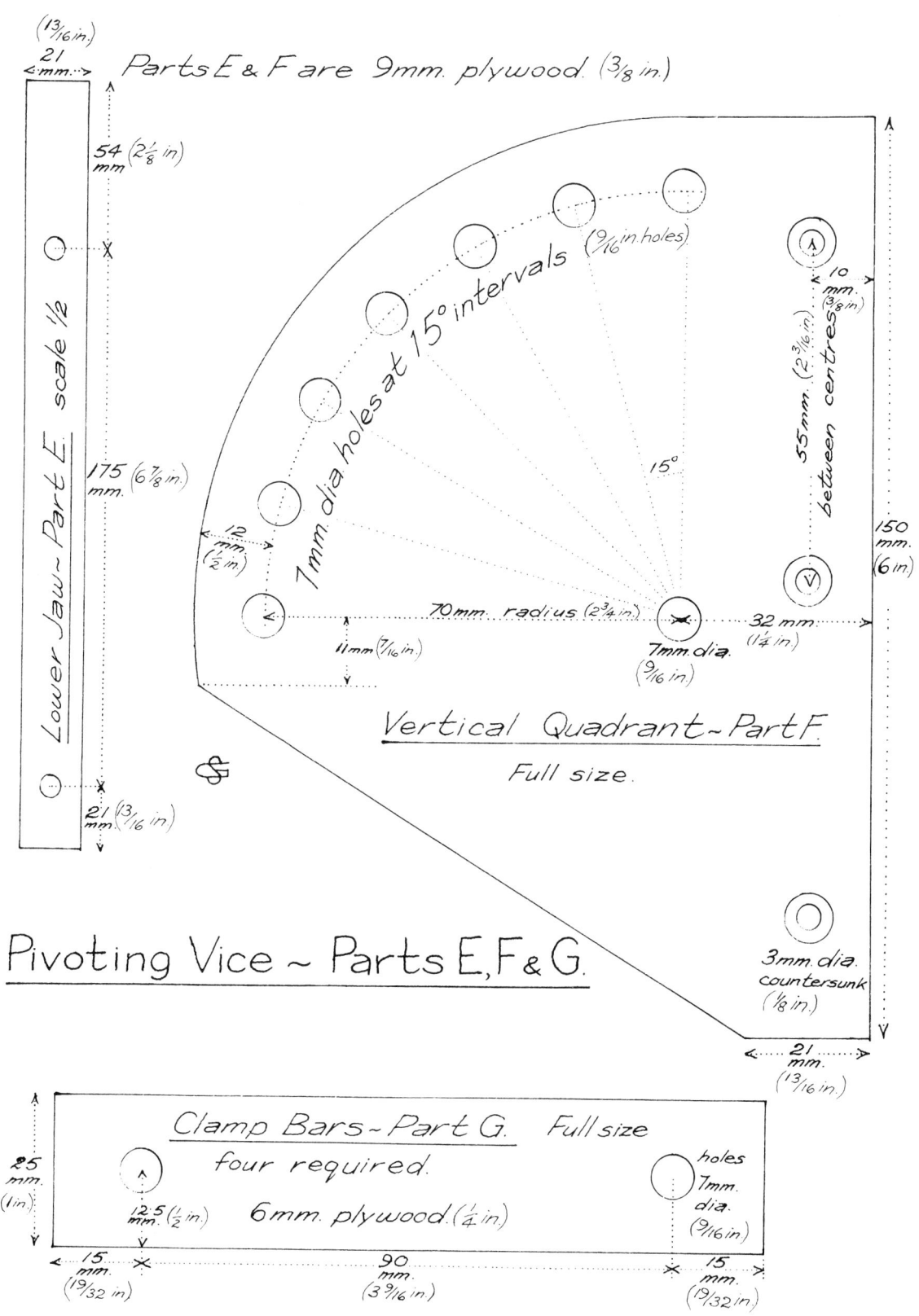

Pivoting Vice ~ Parts E, F & G.

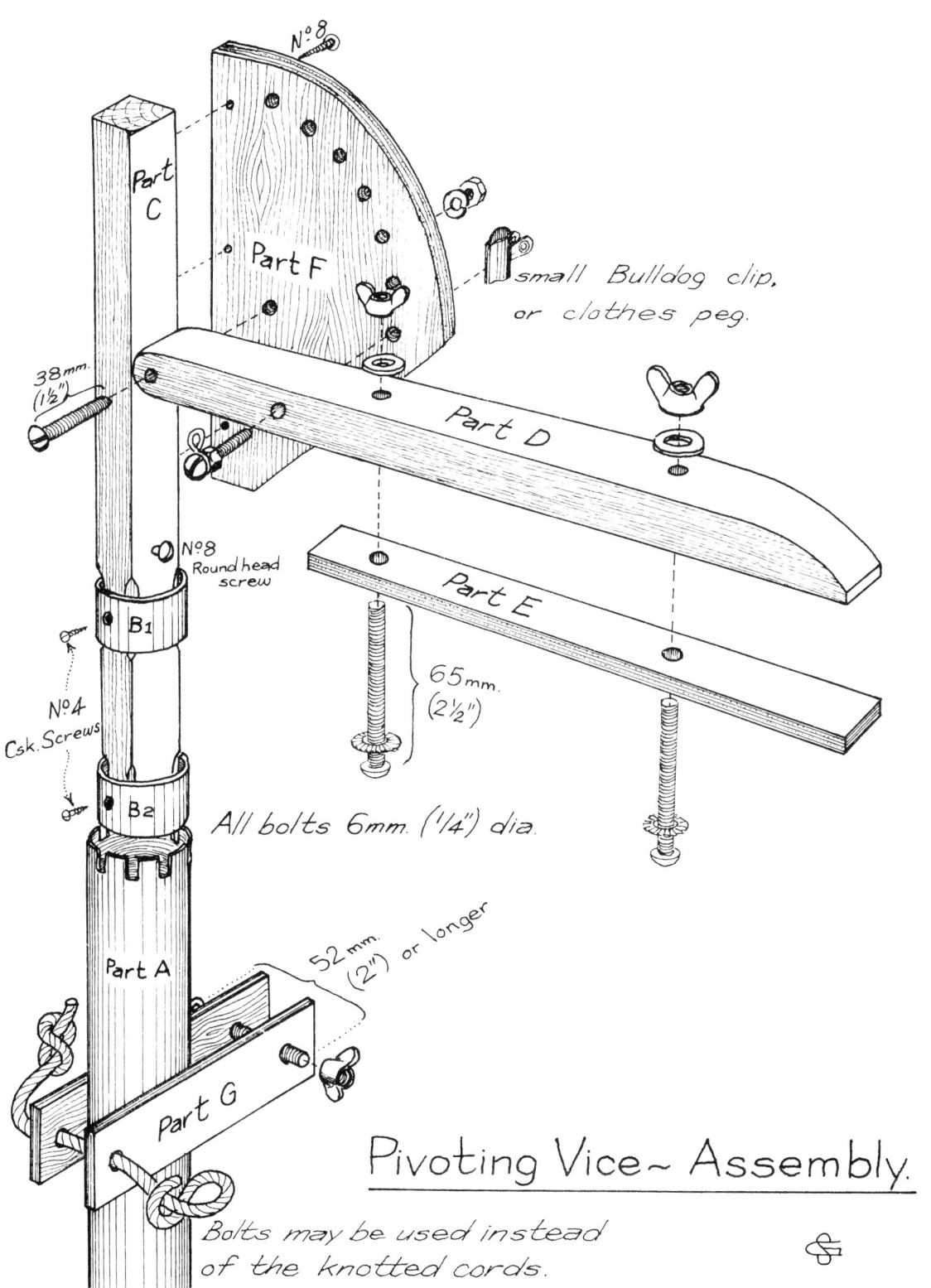

Nº8

Part C

Part F

small Bulldog clip, or clothes peg.

38mm. (1½")

Part D

Nº8 Round head screw

Nº4 Csk. Screws

B₁

B₂

Part E

65mm. (2½")

All bolts 6mm. (¼") dia.

Part A

52mm. (2") or longer

Part G

Pivoting Vice ~ Assembly.

Bolts may be used instead of the knotted cords.

as indicated in the drawing, to accept 6 mm ($\frac{1}{4}$ in.) diameter bolts.

Part E — Lower Jaw of Vice   This Part is a rectangle of 9 mm ($\frac{3}{8}$ in.) plywood, 250 mm x 21 mm ($9\frac{7}{8}$ x $\frac{13}{16}$ in.), drilled with two 6 mm ($\frac{1}{4}$ in.) holes to coincide with the vertical holes in Part D. Two 6 mm x 65 mm ($\frac{1}{4}$ x $2\frac{5}{8}$ in.) bolts are passed upward through the holes in the Lower Jaw and then through the Upper Jaw, being secured on top of Part D with wing nuts above washers.

Part F — Vertical Quadrant   Cut from 9 mm ($\frac{3}{8}$ in.) plywood to the shape and dimensions indicated in the drawing, this Part provides the link between the Pivoting Upright — Part C — and the vertically tilting Upper Jaw of the vice — Part D. The Quadrant is screwed to the Pivoting Upright with three countersunk No. 8 screws. The Upper Jaw — Part D — is attached by a 6 mm ($\frac{1}{4}$ in.) diameter x 38 mm ($1\frac{1}{2}$ in.) bolt passed through the hole in the rounded end of Part D and the central hole in Part F, then secured at the other side of the Quadrant by a lock washer and nut. Part D now pivots vertically about the bolt and against the Quadrant. It can be locked into one of seven positions by passing either a 6 mm x 38 mm ($\frac{1}{4}$ x $1\frac{1}{2}$ in.) bolt or a similar length of rod through the remaining hole in Part D and one of the seven holes spaced at 15° intervals around the radius of the Quadrant. The locking pin or bolt may be secured by means of a Bulldog paper clip or a clothes peg clipped to the free end of the pin. It is convenient to attach the pin and its securing clip to each end of a suitable length of cord, passed through the Quadrant, or a screw eye appropriately positioned. In this way the pin and its clip cannot fall out of reach or get lost.

Parts G — Clamp Bars   Four of these are required to make two clamps, by means of which the completed assembly can be secured to one leg of a chair, or any other suitable spar that may be convenient. The Clamp Bars are simple rectangles of 6 mm ($\frac{1}{4}$ in.) plywood, 120 mm x 25 mm ($3\frac{3}{4}$ x 1 in.), with holes drilled 15 mm ($\frac{5}{8}$ in.) from each end to accept 6 mm ($\frac{1}{4}$ in.) dia x 52 mm (2 in.) bolts with wing nuts. The Clamps are positioned around the socket tube — Part A — and around the chair leg or spar, as far apart as possible. Ideally the chair leg and Socket Tube should be hard up against each other when the nuts of the Clamp bolts are tightened, so that the Socket Tube is held firmly upright on all sides. If this device is to be regularly or permanently fitted to the same chair, the cost of one pair of bolts may be saved by replacing one bolt on each clamp by a short length of cord, with knots in each end, the distance between them being approximately that of the diameter of the Socket Tube.

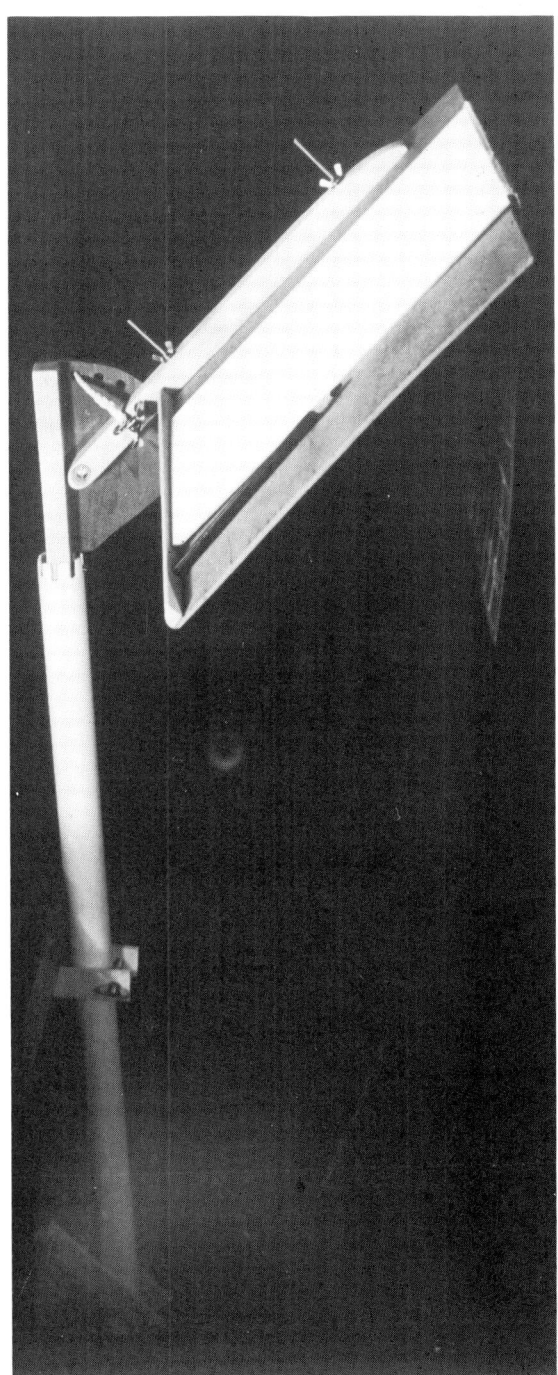

Pivoting Vice with a small Desk Attachment

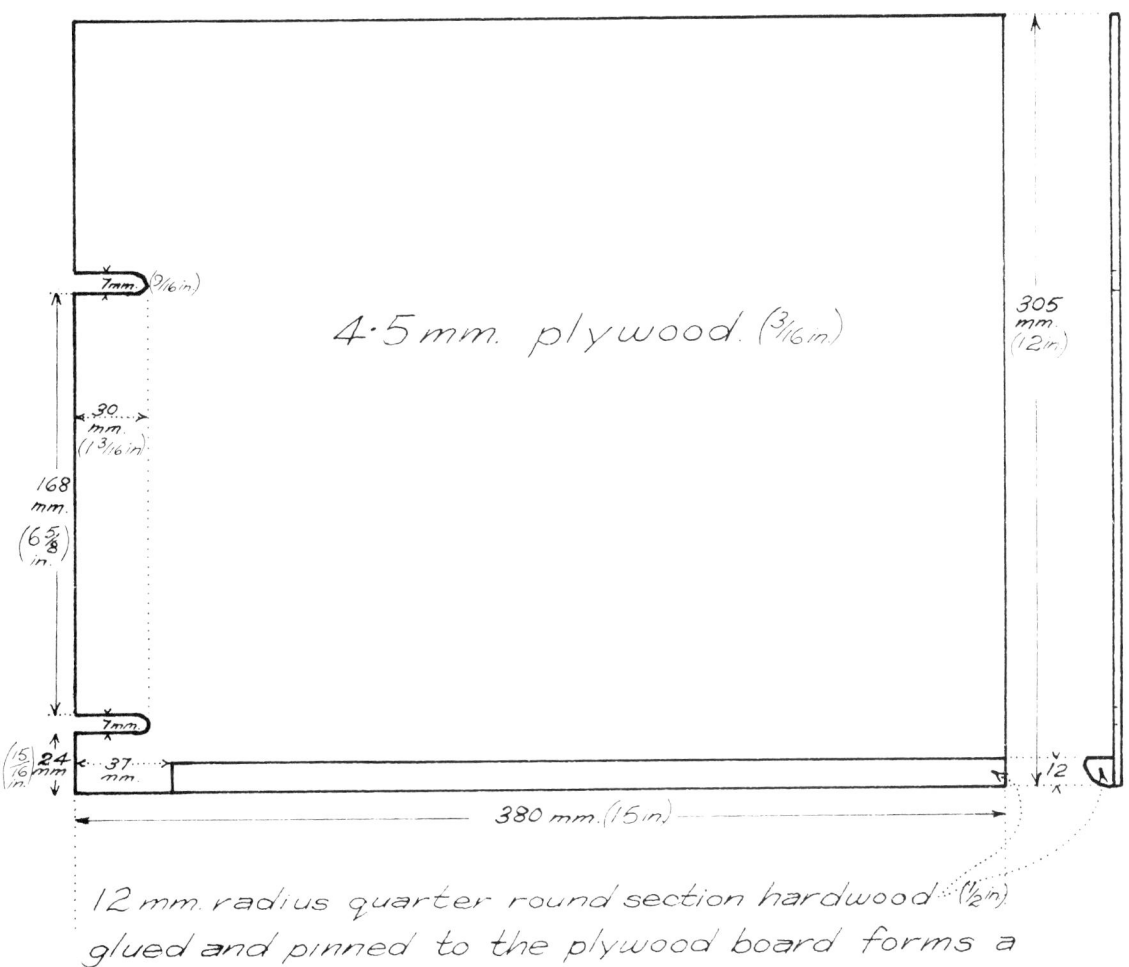

7mm (9/16 in)

4·5mm. plywood. (3/16 in)

305 mm (12 in)

30 mm (1 3/16 in)

168 mm (6 5/8 in)

7mm

(5/16 in) 24mm

37 mm

12

380 mm. (15 in)

12 mm. radius quarter round section hardwood (1/2 in)
glued and pinned to the plywood board forms a
resting rail.

This desk is designed to be held in the Pivoting
Vice. As drawn, the Vice jaws would hold the
desk along its left edge, slotted to pass the
bolts; suitable for a right handed user.

A Small Desk Attachment.

HOLDERS FOR DRINKS

There are so many different shapes and sizes of drinking vessels available that it is not possible to produce a simple design of holder to accommodate all of them. Two very simple, similar — but significantly different — designs of drinks holder are offered here, the first being suited to glasses, tumblers, beakers and mugs, having their height substantially greater than their diameter. This design is

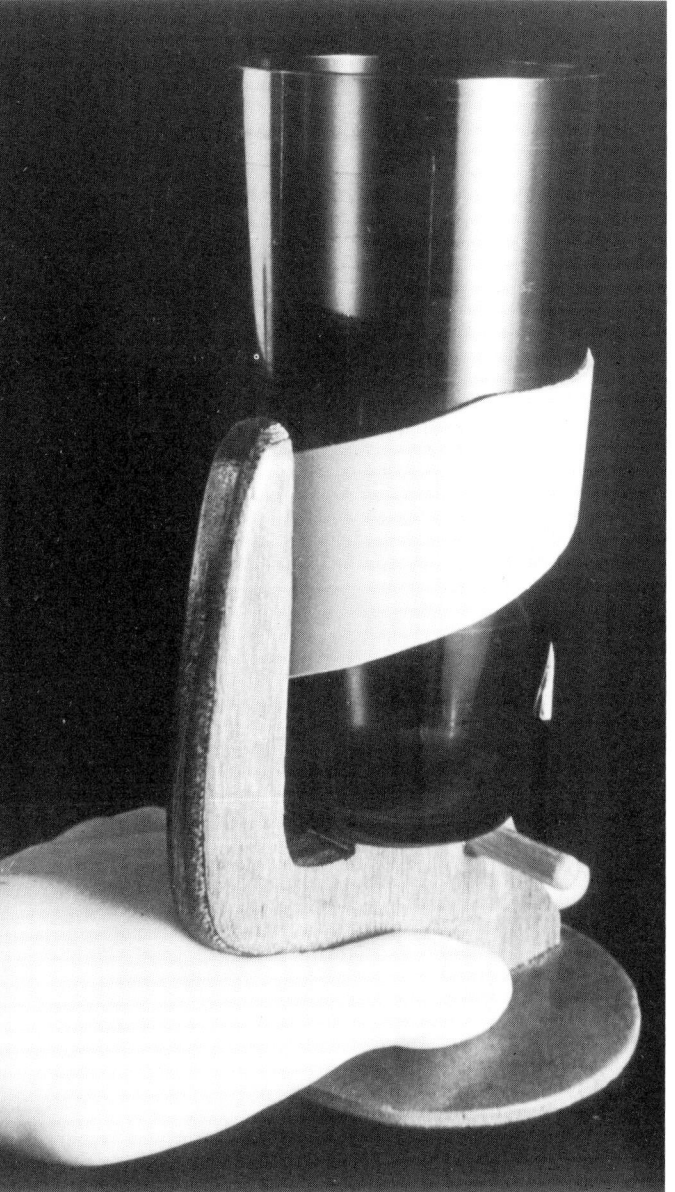

Holder I. The Second design, II, is suited to cups, mugs and glasses, the diameter of which approaches or is greater than their height.

Both designs are intended to provide a means whereby the possessor of weak, stiff or crippled hands can conveniently lift a normal drinking vessel and replace it without help from others. It does not matter whether a cup or mug being used has a handle; if it has, the handle may be ignored, or used by the other hand to steady the vessel. The actual lifting is done by placing the fingers of the lifting hand on each side of the holder, with the palm upward. The shaped Upright part of the holder fits into the palm of the hand comfortably, and enables the weight of the drink to be taken mainly in the palm of the hand, whilst the cross-bar provides a stabilising lever for the fingers. If preferred, an alternative method of holding the Upright is with the palm of the hand facing downward, the thumb placed on one side of the Upright and the fingers on the other side; the Holder is then raised in much the same manner as a wine glass held by the stem would be.

Both designs of holder are most efficient used with drinking vessels having approximately vertical sides, but design I will accommodate more taper in the vessel than will design II. The conventional old-fashioned shape of teacup, like an inverted dome, should not be used in these holders.

The part of both holders which actually grasps the drinking vessel is made from standard plastic pipe, of a type readily available in retail handyman and hardware shops, primarily for rain water drainage. The part is easily washable, so it is not necessary for the drinking vessel to be removed from the holder to be washed on every occasion it is used. Obviously it is desirable that this should be done at regular and fairly frequent intervals, but it could not be done easily by a sufferer from the kind of disability requiring the use of this aid.

It must be understood by the user that the PVC plastic used in this type of water pipe is liable to distort at temperatures approaching boiling point. It is not desirable, therefore, to pour very hot drinks direct into vessels in these holders. Put a little cold milk in before pouring fresh tea or coffee, and be particularly careful with hot soup, which can be even hotter than boiling water.

Holder I with tumbler

A Holder for Drinks I.

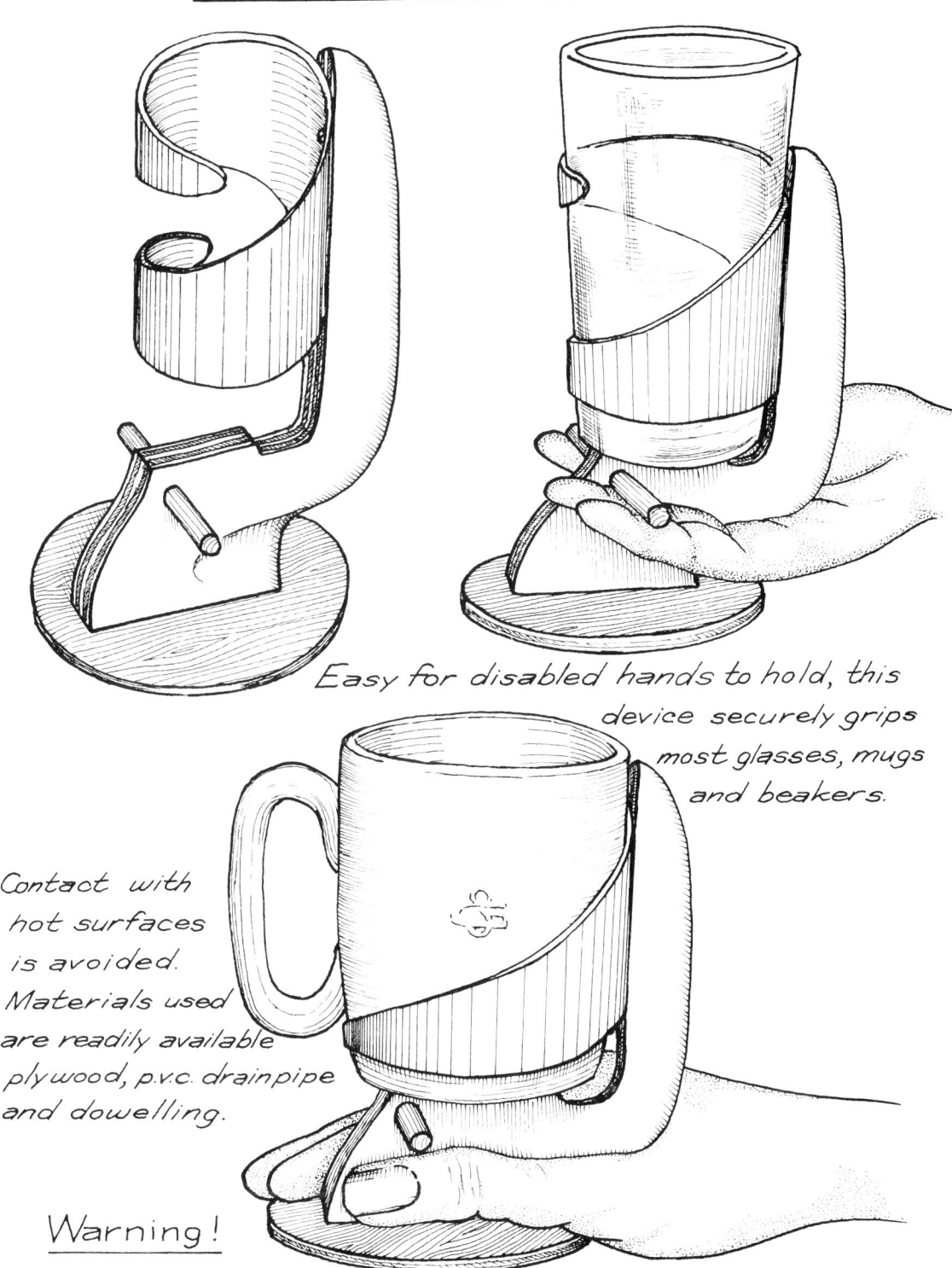

Easy for disabled hands to hold, this device securely grips most glasses, mugs and beakers.

Contact with hot surfaces is avoided. Materials used are readily available plywood, p.v.c. drainpipe and dowelling.

Warning!

The p.v.c. will distort at temperatures near boiling point so add a little cold before pouring in boiling liquid.

The second type of holder, design II, is to be preferred for hot drinks, because the wall thickness of the pipe used for this sleeve is substantially greater than the taller holder's sleeve in design I.

Components and assembly

There are only four components in either of these holders, a Base, an Upright, a Sleeve and a Cross-bar. The methods of cutting and assembly are the same in both cases.

Part R — Base This is simply a disc of 3 mm ($\frac{1}{8}$ in.) plywood, with two holes drilled through it, countersunk underneath, to accept No. 6 x 20 mm ($\frac{3}{4}$ in.) screws, preferably brass, which hold the Base and Upright together.

Part P — Sleeve Note that the principle of the sleeve is basically the same as that of the split spiral mentioned earlier. In the taller holder, design I, this is made from PVC pipe of 54 mm ($2\frac{1}{8}$ in.) outside diameter, whereas in the shorter holder, design II, it is of approximately 68 mm ($2\frac{11}{16}$ in.) outside diameter and a substantially greater wall thickness. To mark the plastic pipe prior to cutting, trace the appropriate diagram provided onto a piece of paper and then wrap the paper around the tube, holding it in place with adhesive tape or elastic bands. Prick through the paper and into the tube at intervals along the cutting lines, using the point of a needle. The paper is then removed from the tube, and the pricked marks can be joined up to provide a guide line, using a chinagraph pencil or felt tip pen. A piercing saw, coping saw or tenon saw can be used to cut along the marked lines, a little at a time, holding the pipe in a vice and turning it repeatedly. Finally, two holes, 20 mm ($\frac{3}{4}$ in.) apart and countersunk on the inside, are drilled through the back of the sleeve on the centreline, through which the screws holding the Sleeve to the Upright are placed.

Part Q — Upright This part may be cut from either 9 mm ($\frac{3}{8}$ in.) or 12 mm ($\frac{1}{2}$ in.) plywood, in accordance with the respective drawings. Pilot holes for screws — preferably brass — are drilled into the inner face of the Upright and into the underneath of it. Finally a hole of 6 mm ($\frac{1}{4}$ in.) diameter is drilled through the Upright into which the Cross-bar is glued centrally.

The Cross-Bar 60 to 65 mm ($2\frac{3}{8}$ to $2\frac{9}{16}$ in.) of 6 mm ($\frac{1}{4}$ in.) diameter dowelling is glued on the centreline through the Upright, projecting an equal amount on each side of it.

Finishing

The woodwork of the Holders should be well sealed, preferably with at least two coats of polyurethane sealer, and then either varnished or painted. The better the final finish produced the easier it will be to keep the Holder clean, which is a matter of some importance in an aid of this kind.

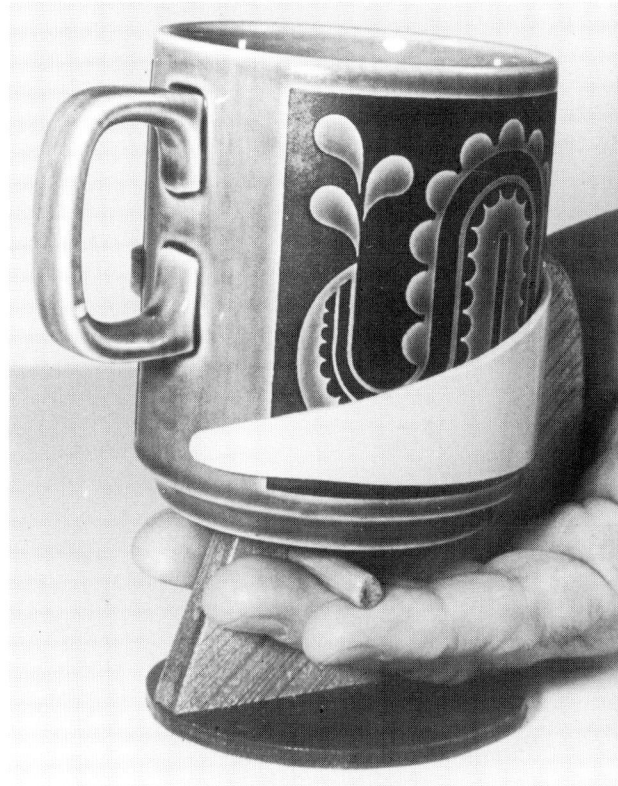

Drinks Holder II with a Hornsea mug

A Holder for Drinks. I.

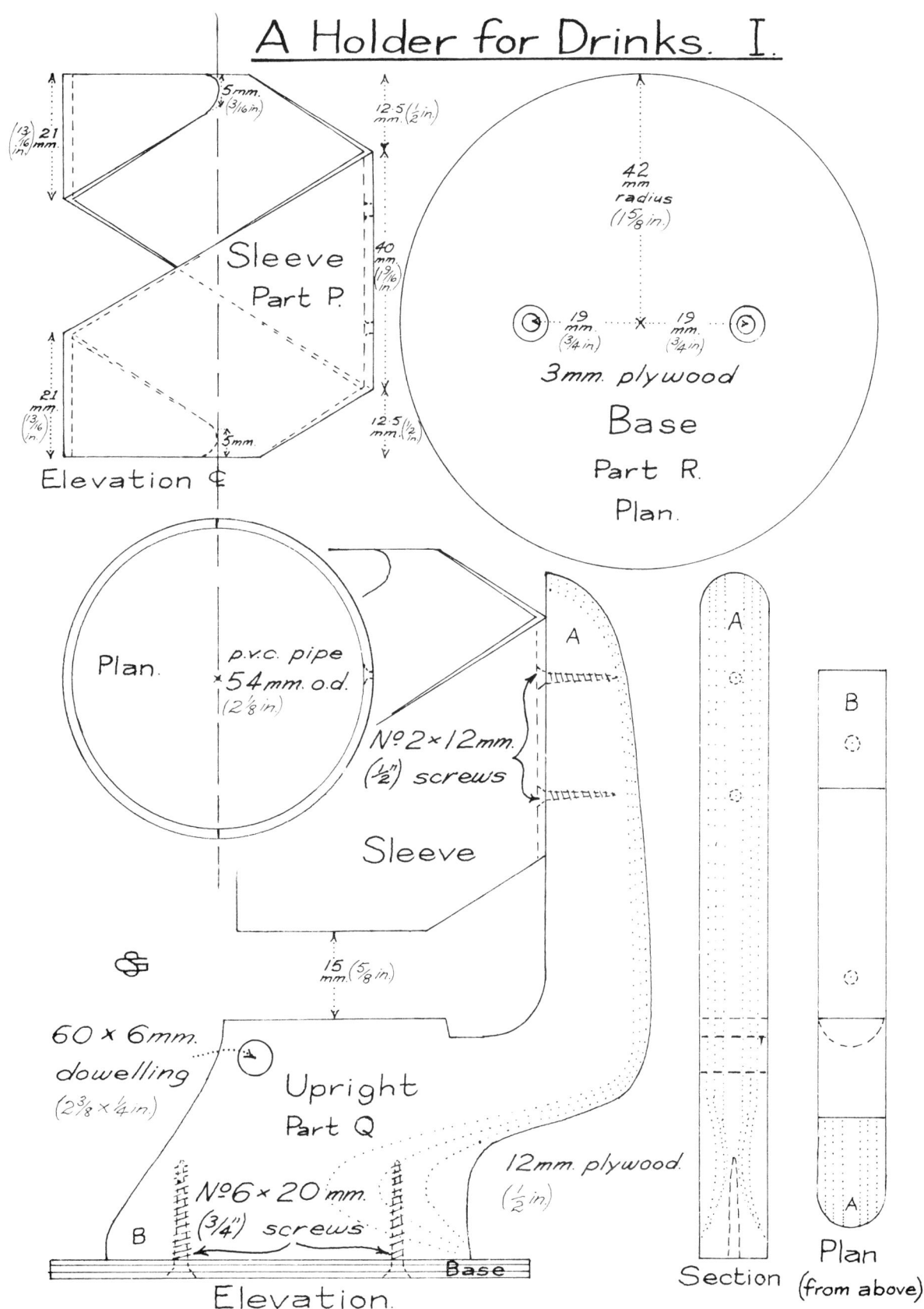

Sleeve
Part P.

Elevation ₵

5mm.
(3/16 in.)

21 mm. (13/16 in.)

40 mm. (1 9/16 in.)

12.5 mm. (1/2 in.)

21 mm. (13/16 in.)

12.5 mm. (1/2 in.)

42 mm. radius (1 5/8 in.)

19 mm. (3/4 in.)   19 mm. (3/4 in.)

3mm. plywood

Base
Part R.
Plan.

Plan.

p.v.c. pipe
54mm. o.d.
(2 1/8 in.)

Nº 2 × 12mm.
(1/2") screws

Sleeve

15 mm. (5/8 in.)

60 × 6mm.
dowelling
(2 3/8 × 1/4 in.)

Upright
Part Q

Nº 6 × 20 mm.
(3/4") screws

12mm. plywood
(1/2 in.)

Base

Elevation.

A

A

Section

B

A

Plan
(from above)

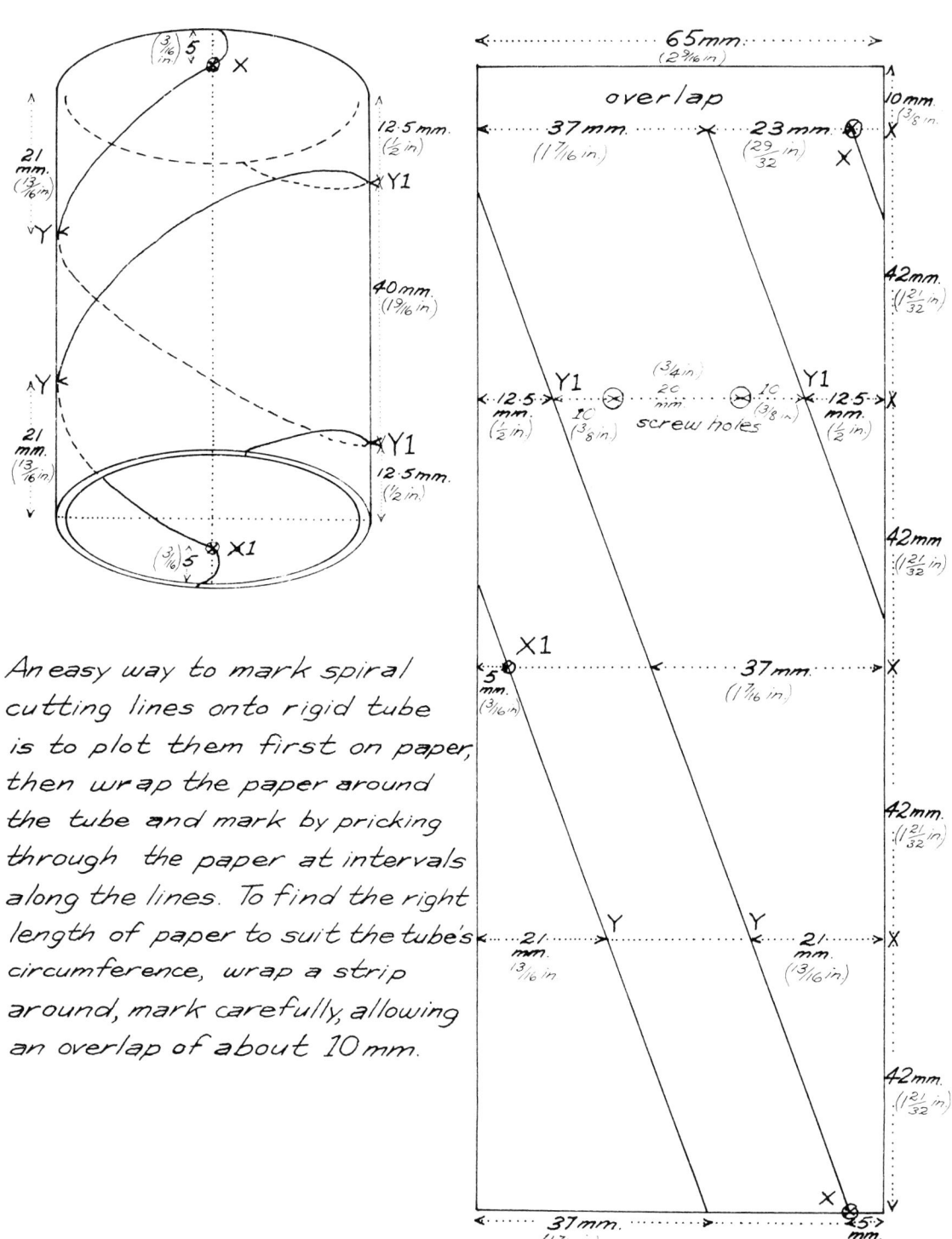

An easy way to mark spiral
cutting lines onto rigid tube
is to plot them first on paper,
then wrap the paper around
the tube and mark by pricking
through the paper at intervals
along the lines. To find the right
length of paper to suit the tube's
circumference, wrap a strip
around, mark carefully, allowing
an overlap of about 10 mm.

I. Sleeve - Part P. Marking tube to be cut.

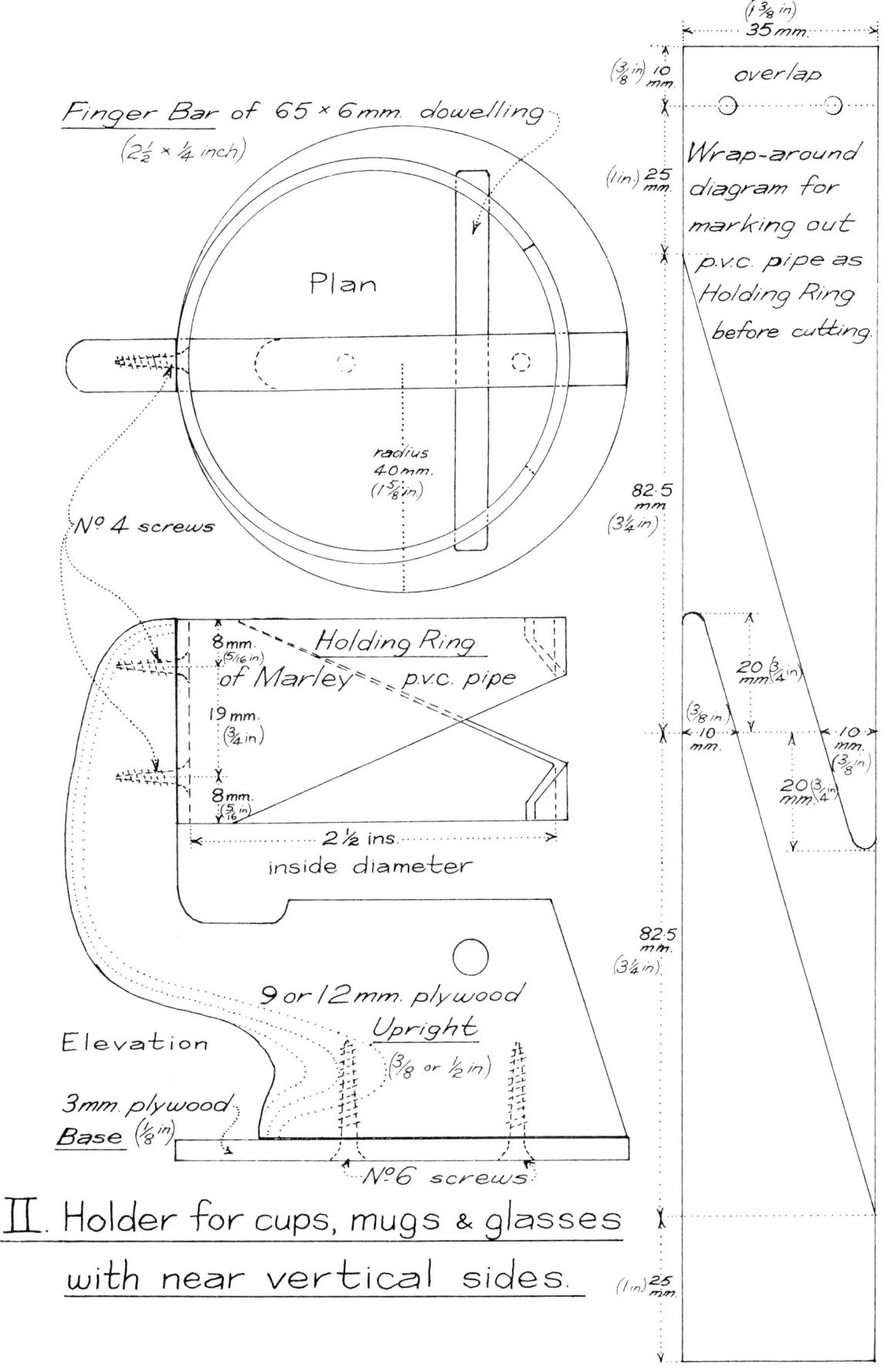

Finger Bar of 65 × 6mm. dowelling
(2½ × ¼ inch)

Plan

radius
40 mm.
(1⅝in)

Nº 4 screws

8mm.
(5/16 in)

Holding Ring
of Marley   p.v.c. pipe

19 mm.
(¾ in)

8 mm.
(5/16)

2 ½ ins.
inside diameter

9 or 12 mm. plywood
Upright
(⅜ or ½ in)

Elevation

3mm. plywood
Base (⅛ in)

Nº 6 screws

Ⅱ. Holder for cups, mugs & glasses
with near vertical sides.

(1⅜ in)
35 mm

(⅜ in) 10 mm

overlap

(1 in) 25 mm

Wrap-around
diagram for
marking out
p.v.c. pipe as
Holding Ring
before cutting.

82·5
mm
(3¼ in)

20 (¾ in)
mm

(⅜ in)
10
mm

10
mm
(⅜ in)

20 (¾ in)
mm

82·5
mm
(3¼ in)

(1 in) 25 mm

SCISSORS OPERATOR

The purpose of this device is to provide a means whereby a pair of scissors may be used without being held in the hand and without the hand being flexed. Pressure on the cross-bar of the device closes the scissors and an elastic band acts as a spring to open them again.

Materials

122 x 132 mm (4.8 x 5.2 in.) of 12 mm ($\frac{1}{2}$ in.) thick plywood.

150 x 60 mm (6 x 2$\frac{3}{8}$ in.) of 4 mm ($\frac{3}{16}$ in.) thick plywood.

75 x 6 mm (3 x $\frac{1}{4}$ in.) diameter dowelling.

1 roofing bolt 6 mm ($\frac{1}{4}$ in.) dia. x 30 mm (1$\frac{1}{4}$ in.) with washer and butterfly nut.

1 countersunk bolt 6 mm ($\frac{1}{4}$ in.) dia. x 28 mm (1$\frac{1}{8}$ in.) with lock washer and nut.

70 x 35 mm (2$\frac{3}{4}$ x 1$\frac{3}{8}$ in.) aluminium or brass sheet about 1 mm (20 gauge S.W.G.) thick.

70 x 40 mm (2$\frac{3}{4}$ x 1$\frac{9}{16}$ in.) rubber from tyre inner tube.

washer 30 mm (1$\frac{3}{16}$ in.) dia. of rubber from inner tube.

2 No. 10 raised head or round head screws x 38 mm (1$\frac{1}{2}$ in.).

2 No. 6 countersunk head screws x 16 to 20 mm ($\frac{5}{8}$ to $\frac{3}{4}$ in.).

one or two elastic bands about 75 mm (3 in.) long.

Components

Part A – Lever is traced onto and cut from 12 mm ($\frac{1}{2}$ in.) plywood and drilled with two 6 mm ($\frac{1}{4}$ in.) holes — one at the end, for the dowelling cross-bar, and one at the centre for the countersunk pivot bolt. Pilot holes for the two No. 10 screws are drilled at the end furthest from the cross-bar.

Part B – Upright is traced onto and cut from 12 mm ($\frac{1}{2}$ in.) plywood, then drilled with a countersunk 6 mm ($\frac{1}{4}$ in.) hole for the countersunk pivot bolt. A 6 mm ($\frac{1}{4}$ in.) wide curved slot is cut through the top projection to accommodate the roofing bolt and allow adjustment. Two Pilot holes for the No. 6 screws are drilled into the bottom edge.

Part C – Base is made from the rectangular piece of 4 mm ($\frac{3}{16}$ in.) plywood, with the corners rounded off. Two countersunk holes are drilled in the underside for the two No. 6 screws.

Part D is cut from the sheet metal, drilled with a 6 mm ($\frac{1}{4}$ in.) hole, and the upper edge is hammered over to form a lip.

Part E is a rubber washer about 30 mm (1$\frac{1}{4}$ in.) in diameter with a 6 mm ($\frac{1}{4}$ in.) hole.

Part F is a facing piece made from the inner tube rubber and glued to the upper part of Part B — the Upright.

Assembly

Apply glue to the centre of the dowelling Cross-bar and fix it in position through the hole in Part A. Apply glue to the lower edge of Part B and screw Part C to it with the two No. 6 screws. Screw the two No. 10 screws in to Part A, leaving about 24 mm (1 in.) of each standing clear above the surface. File down the protruding points of these screws until they are flush with the surface. Pass the countersunk pivot bolt through the hole in Part B, then through the central hole in Part A and secure it in place with the nut and lock washer.

Pass the roofing bolt through the hole in Part D, through the rubber washer Part E, then through the thumb hole of a pair of scissors and finally through the slot in Parts F and B, securing it with the butterfly nut and washer. The finger hole of the pair of scissors should be placed either over the upper No. 10 screw or over both of these screws. (Experiment will show which alternative works best with a particular pair of scissors.) Position the scissors so that their pivot lies as close as possible to the pivot bolt head. Adjust Part D and the securing bolt in its slot so that the scissors can be fully closed, then tighten the butterfly nut to hold the pair of scissors rigidly in place.

Operating the lever should now open and close the scissors easily, and placing the elastic band between the butterfly nut and the Cross-bar provides enough spring to open the scissors after each cut. It may be necessary to use more than one elastic band if the scissors are stiff.

Using the Scissors Operator

Operating the device is simplicity itself, once it is properly adjusted, but it is important that the base is firmly positioned. Ideally the base is screwed or clamped to a working surface, but alternatively a layer of non-slip material, such as inner tube rubber, may be glued to the underside of the base. The base

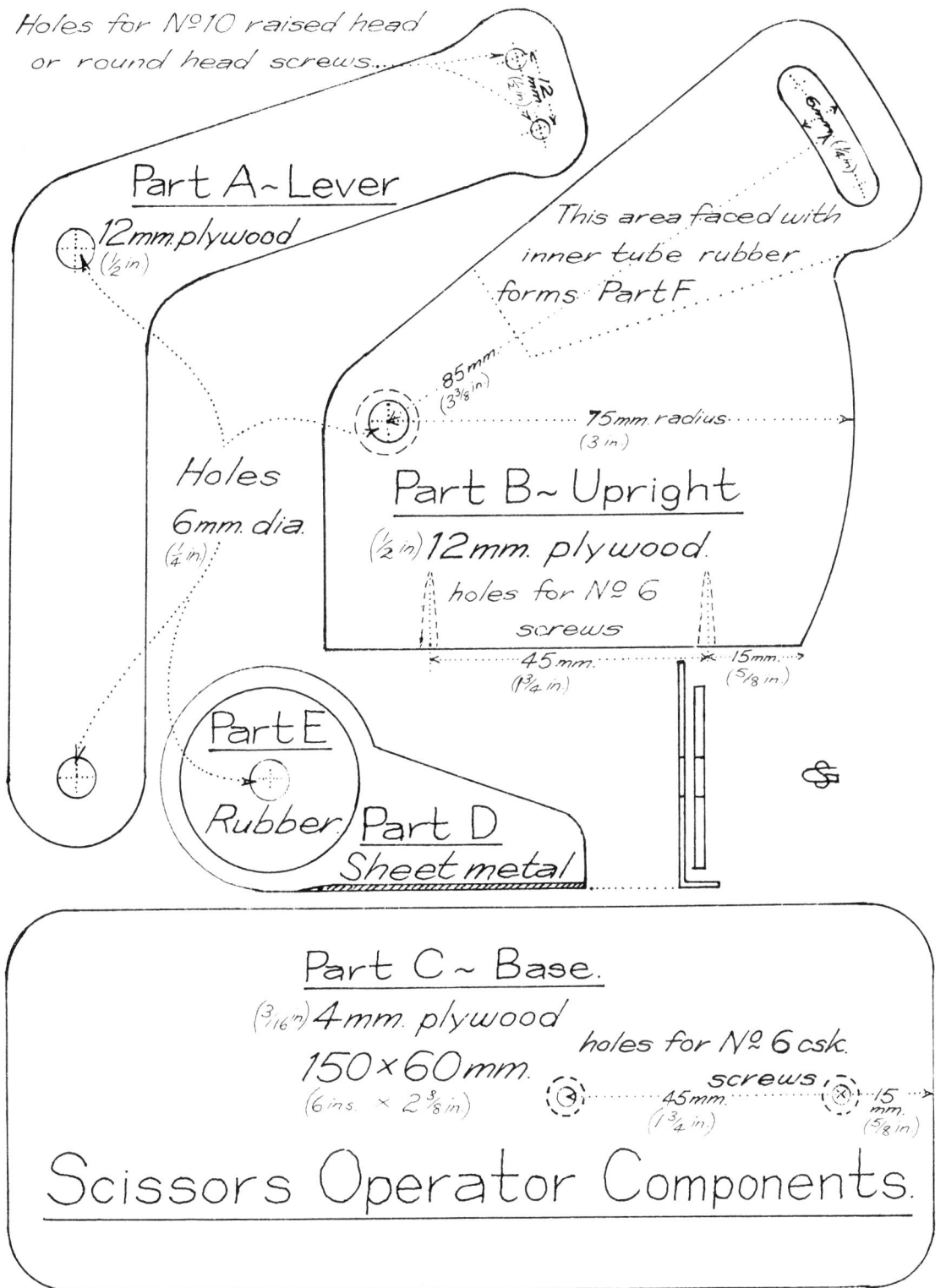

Holes for Nº 10 raised head
or round head screws...

Part A ~ Lever

12 mm. plywood
(½ in)

This area faced with
inner tube rubber
forms Part F

Holes

6 mm. dia.
(¼ in)

85 mm.
(3⅜ in)

75 mm. radius
(3 in)

Part B ~ Upright

(½ in) 12 mm. plywood

holes for Nº 6
screws

45 mm.
(1¾ in)

15 mm.
(⅝ in)

Part E

Rubber. **Part D**

Sheet metal

Part C ~ Base.

(3/16 in) 4 mm. plywood

150 × 60 mm.
(6 ins. × 2⅜ in)

holes for Nº 6 csk.
screws

45 mm.
(1¾ in)

15
mm.
(⅝ in)

Scissors Operator Components.

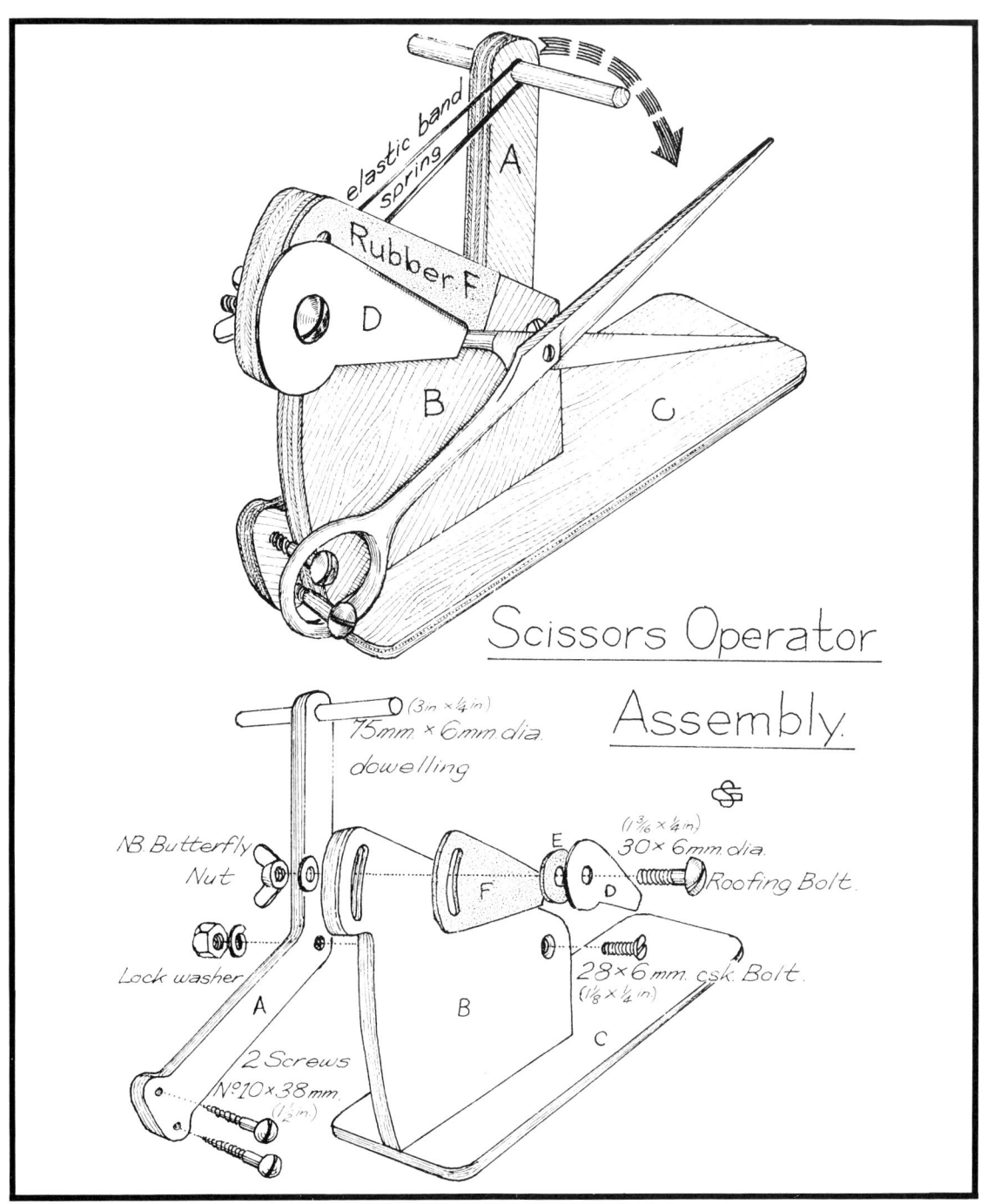

elastic band
spring

Rubber F

A

D

B

C

Scissors Operator

Assembly.

(3 in × ¼ in)
75mm × 6mm dia.
dowelling

N.B. Butterfly
Nut

(1 ³⁄₁₆ × ¼ in)
30 × 6mm dia.
Roofing Bolt.

E

F

D

Lock washer

28 × 6 mm. csk. Bolt.
(1⅛ × ¼ in)

A

B

C

2 Screws
Nº 10 × 38 mm.
(1½ in)

may be made larger and of heavier material if the extra cost is acceptable or a suitable offcut is available.

Cutting with this device will be found easiest if the lower point of the pair of scissors is close to the base. This enables the user to feed the material being cut along the base and between the blades without having to hold it up above the working surface.

Operating devices of this kind can be made to suit any pair of scissors, with slight adjustment of the dimensions, but the design, as it is drawn here, will fit the great majority of working size scissors, up to and including paper hanger's scissors.

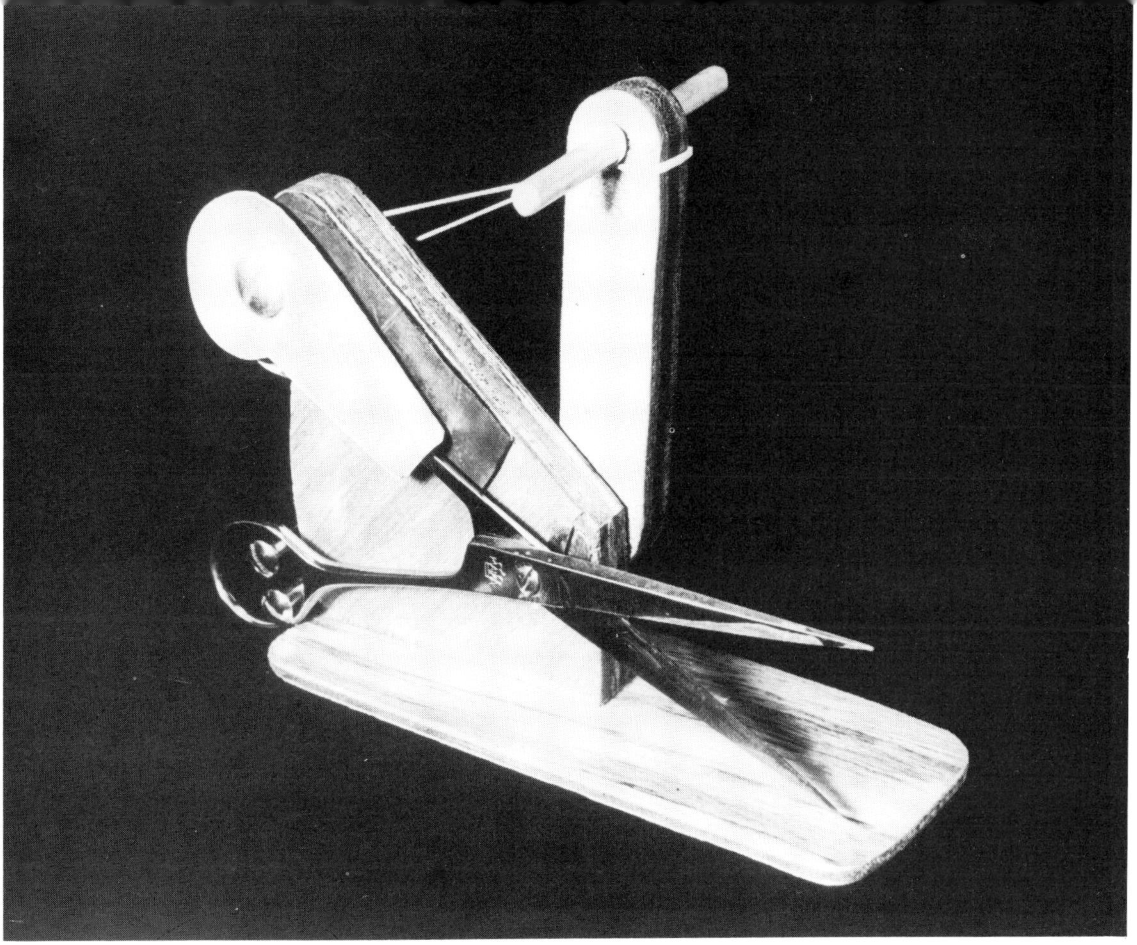

Scissors Operator — front and back

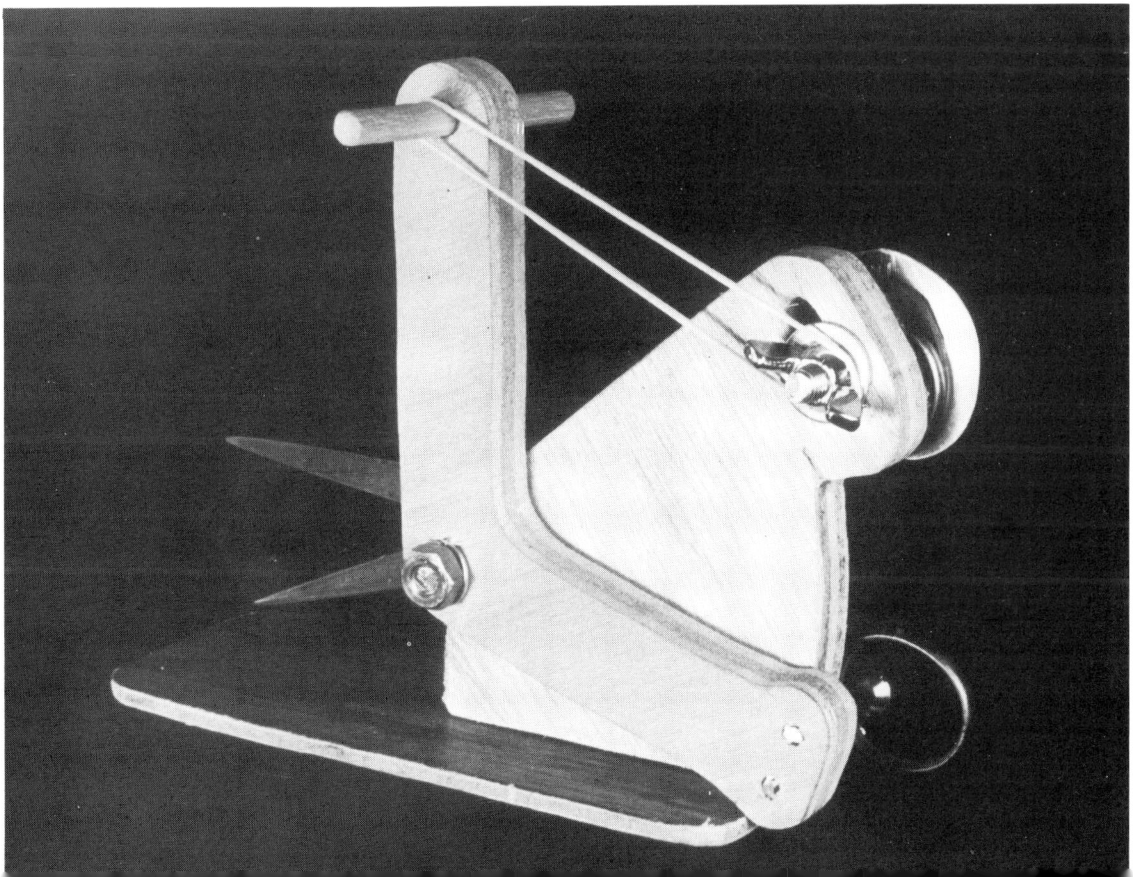

WHEELCHAIR POCKET

It seems the epitome of insult added to injury that many a man who has been deprived of the use of his legs is also deprived of the use of his pockets. The reason for this is that wheelchairs, built to pass through doors of standard width, are, of necessity, a little narrow in the seat and do not allow the occupant much room for manoevering to reach his pockets. The Wheelchair Pocket was designed and made in response to the plea of a frustrated pipe smoker, who could find no satisfactory stowage for tobacco and pipe. It consists of a simple rectangular box or bag, cut in one piece from denim or duck canvas, which can be folded and glued together with Copydex or a similar latex adhesive, without any necessity for sewing. The Pocket is attached to the wheelchair by means of two strips of webbing secured beneath one arm-rest. Four plastic Meccano nuts and bolts hold the webbing straps and pocket together and this enables the pocket to be removed easily for washing.

Material

Denim or duck canvas 500 x 275 mm (20 x $10\frac{13}{16}$ in.).

Nylon webbing, about 460 mm (18 in.) long x approx. 50 mm (2 in.) wide.

4 bolts with nuts, preferably plastic, 15 x 10 mm ($\frac{5}{8}$ x $\frac{3}{8}$ in.).

Copydex or equivalent glue.

Velcro fastening, approx. 80 x 20 mm (3 x $\frac{3}{4}$ in.).

Construction

Carefully draw the outline and the fold lines of the Pocket on to the denim or canvas. Cut around the outline, then iron the folds in place with a hot iron. Glue down the hems indicated in the plan drawing. Apply Copydex or equivalent to both surfaces being joined, allow a couple of minutes drying time and then press the surfaces together. It is a good idea to have a piece of dowelling, tube or broom handle ready, with which the glued hems and seams can be rolled to apply even pressure. When the hems have been glued, the bottom can be glued to the sides in the same way, and finally the back and sides are glued together, as shown in (3). The only sewing needed is to secure the Velcro fastening strips in place — see (4).

The holes in the Pocket and nylon webbing straps can be cut most easily with a suitable punch but, with care, a sharp craft knife will do the job. The best way of finishing the holes is to use brass eyelets, which are riveted into position with a special punch and die. However, unless such equipment can be borrowed or hired an alternative is necessary, because this equipment is too expensive to buy specially. The edges of the holes in the nylon webbing can be sealed by melting with a hot soldering iron, thus fusing the fibres together. The edges of holes in the denim or canvas can be sealed by applying Copydex glue to them and allowing it to dry thoroughly before use. This can be reinforced with buttonhole stitching if so desired.

Attaching the Pocket to the wheelchair

Most wheel chairs have padded arm-rests, which are secured to a tubular metal frame by means of screws or bolts, entered from underneath. If the screws or bolts holding one of the arm-rests are loosened, that arm-rest can be raised off the frame sufficiently for the ends of the two webbing straps to be tucked through the gap. The arm-rest securing screws then can be tightened up again, so that the webbing is gripped tightly between the arm-rest and frame, thus holding the pocket securely in position.

1. Draw full size and cut out the shape to the given measurements from denim or duck canvas.

2. Apply Copydex to the indicated edges, fold them over and glue down to shaded areas to make secure hems.

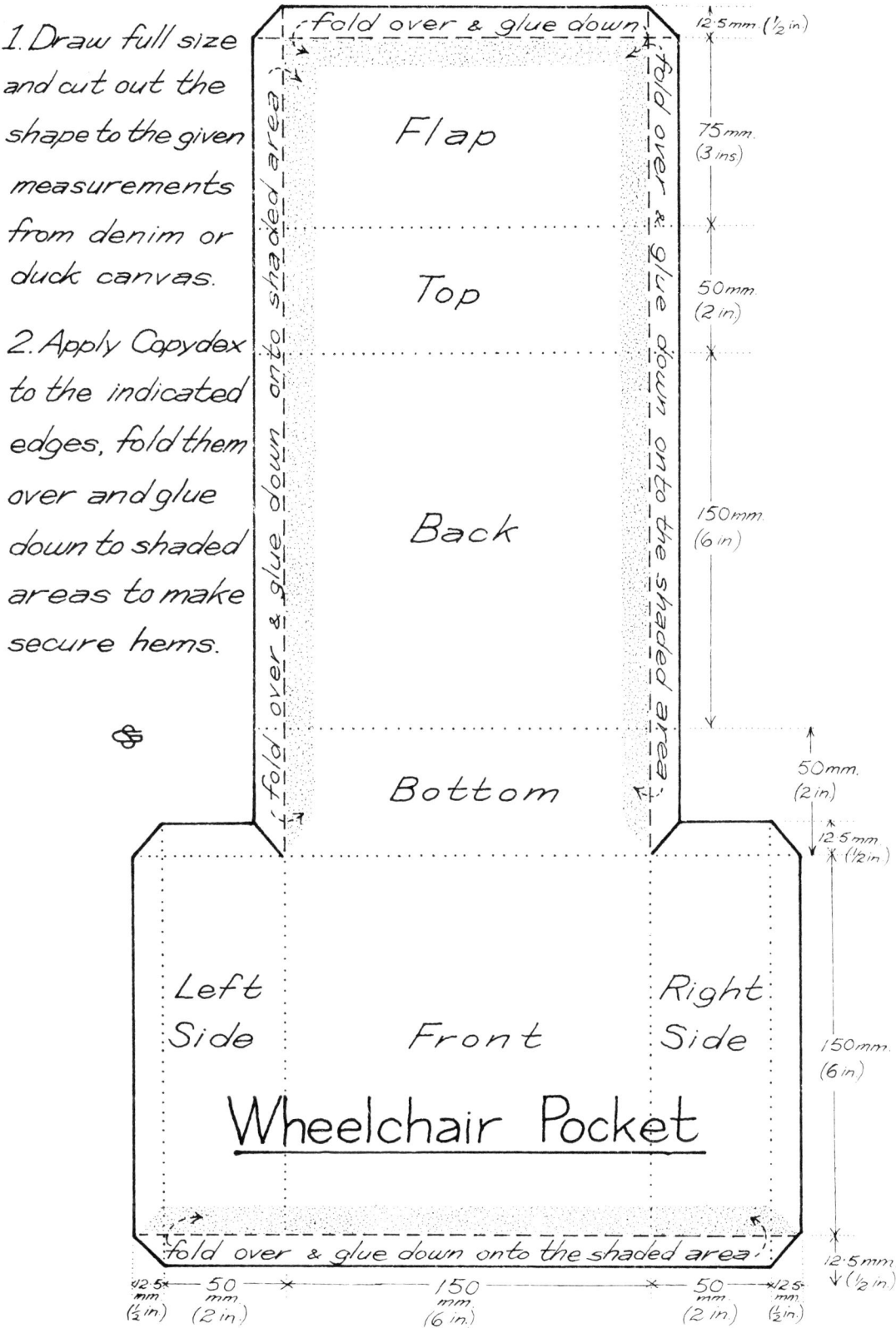

fold over & glue down

Flap

Top

Back

Bottom

fold over & glue down onto shaded area

fold over & glue down onto the shaded area

12.5mm (½ in)

75mm (3 ins)

50mm (2 in)

150mm (6 in)

50mm (2 in)

12.5mm (½ in)

Left Side

Front

Right Side

Wheelchair Pocket

fold over & glue down onto the shaded area

150mm (6 in)

12.5mm (½ in)

12.5 mm (½ in)

50 mm (2 in)

150 mm (6 in)

50 mm (2 in)

12.5 mm (½ in)

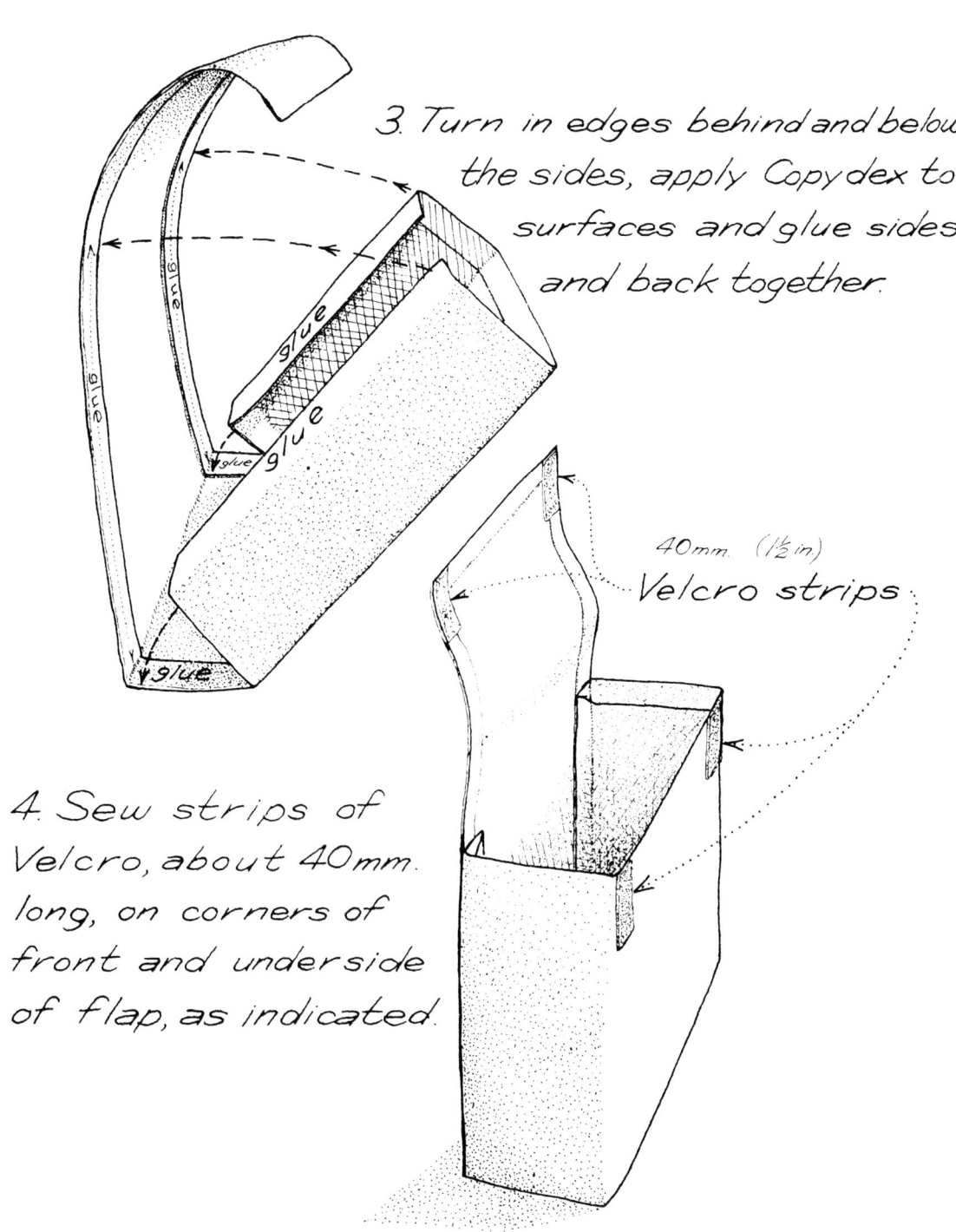

3. Turn in edges behind and below the sides, apply Copydex to surfaces and glue sides and back together.

40mm. (1½ in)
Velcro strips

4. Sew strips of Velcro, about 40mm. long, on corners of front and underside of flap, as indicated.

glue

Wheelchair Pocket. ✧

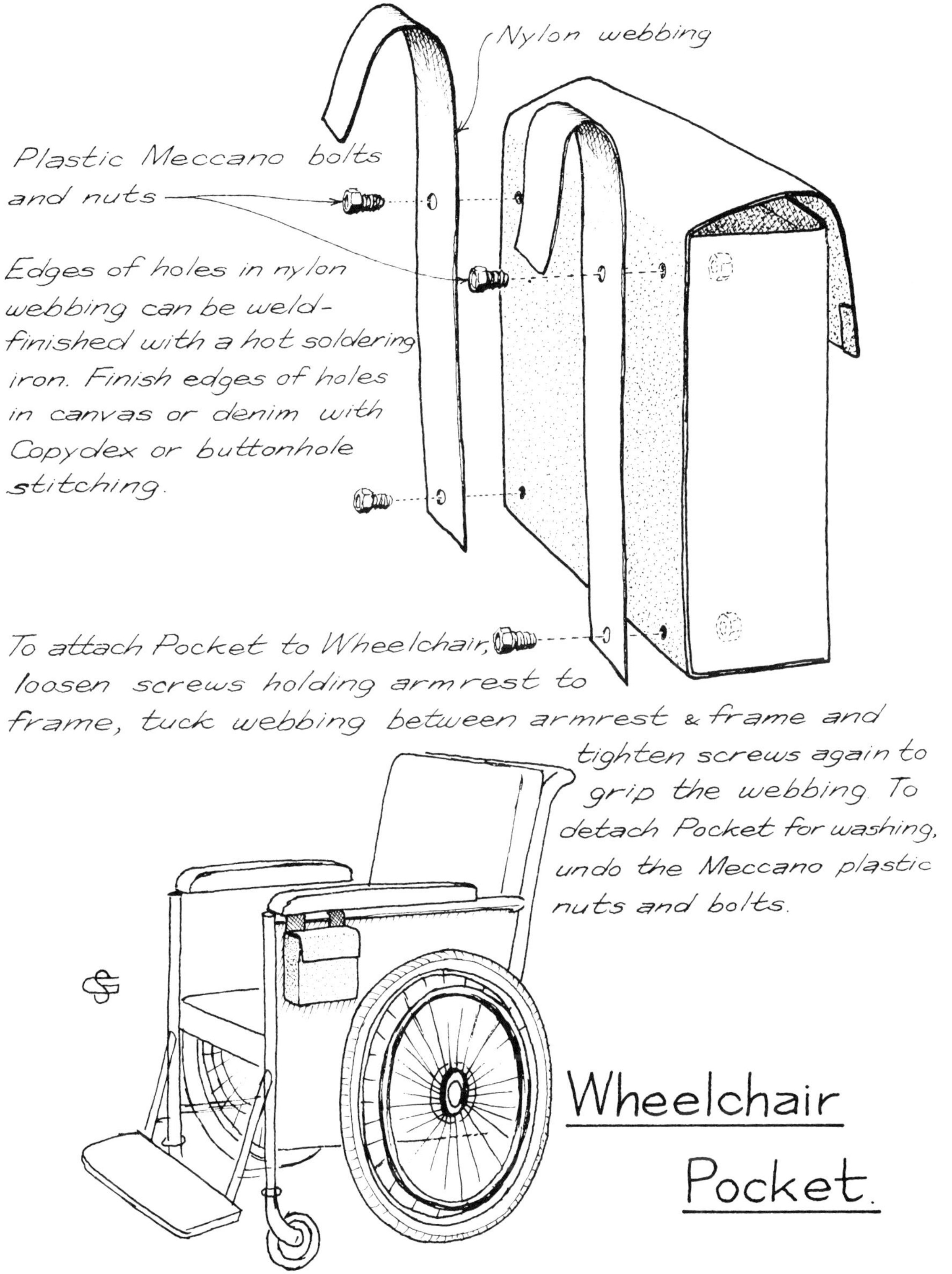

Nylon webbing

Plastic Meccano bolts
and nuts

Edges of holes in nylon
webbing can be weld-
finished with a hot soldering
iron. Finish edges of holes
in canvas or denim with
Copydex or buttonhole
stitching.

To attach Pocket to Wheelchair,
loosen screws holding armrest to
frame, tuck webbing between armrest & frame and
tighten screws again to
grip the webbing. To
detach Pocket for washing,
undo the Meccano plastic
nuts and bolts.

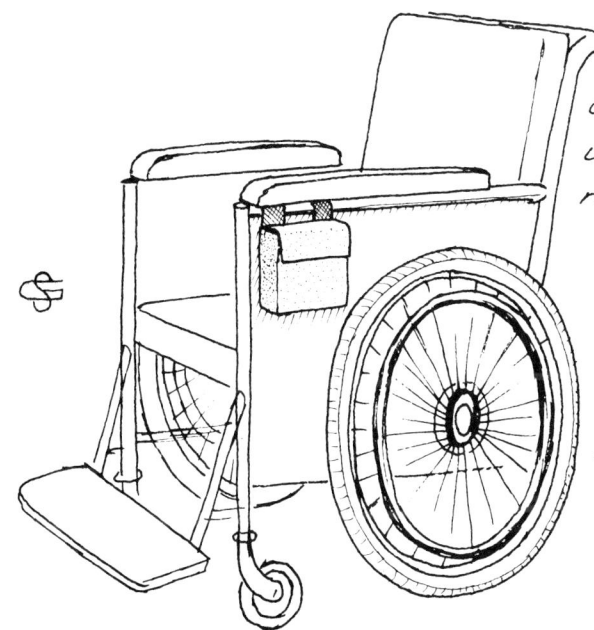

Wheelchair
Pocket.

TEAPOT POURING STAND

It can be both difficult and dangerous for anyone with weak or painful hands or arms to try to lift and pour from a pot full of boiling hot liquid. This Pouring Stand is designed to provide a stable, hinged platform, upon which such a tea or coffee pot may be placed and tilted safely for pouring into cups or mugs. The blind or partially sighted may also find this device helpful.

There are so many different shapes and sizes of teapot, let alone coffee pots and jugs, that it is impractical to expect one design to be suitable for every pot. Nevertheless, the design offered here has been found to suit the great majority of teapots tried out upon it, and many coffee pots too, although it may be advisable to increase the height of the Fences — Parts G — for very tall pots. The design provided here is basically very simple and anyone handy enough to make it at all will be capable of adjusting it to suit a particular size or shape of pot. It may be scaled up horizontally to provide a permanent platform for an electric kettle.

It is necessary to ensure that the pot sits securely on the Platform (Part A), between the Fences and the Handle, with the spout, from which the liquid is poured, projecting forward between the Fences. As the Handle is lifted for pouring, and the Platform tilts forward, the weight of the pot is increasingly transferred onto the Fences. It is, therefore, most important that they are fixed strongly to the Platform, and are of sufficient size to hold the pot securely. It will be noted that the Fences, as designed, have projections at their bases, which fit into slots in the Platform. This not only provides considerable strength, but also has the advantage that the Fences can be fitted and tried out, using cold water, with any particular pot, before they are finally glued into place. Thus any modification which appears desirable can be effected before any irrevocable step in assembly is taken.

Materials

365 x 150 x 9 mm ($14\frac{3}{8}$ x $5\frac{15}{16}$ x $\frac{3}{8}$ in.) plywood.

40 x 20 x 20 mm ($1\frac{9}{16}$ x $\frac{4}{5}$ x $\frac{4}{5}$ in.) hard wood.

120 x 9 mm ($4\frac{3}{4}$ x $\frac{3}{8}$ in.) diameter dowelling.

Two screws approximately 20 mm ($\frac{3}{4}$ in.) long No. 2 or 4 countersunk.

Two panel pins about 15 mm ($\frac{5}{8}$ in.) long.

Wood glue.

Components

Refer to the drawings throughout. Note that Parts A, B, E, F and G are all cut from 9 mm ($\frac{3}{8}$ in.) plywood.

Part A — Platform is what the teapot actually stands upon. It has two slots cut through it near the front, into which the Fences — Parts G — are eventually fitted. Two countersunk holes for No. 2 or 4 screws are drilled through the front, countersunk from the top.

Part B — Handle is pinned and glued in position at the rear and underside of the Platform — Part A.

Parts C — Bearings are two 20 mm ($\frac{4}{5}$ in.) cubes of hardwood, drilled centrally to accept 9 mm ($\frac{3}{8}$ in.) diameter dowelling. A pilot hole for a 15 mm ($\frac{5}{8}$ in.) long No. 2 or 4 screw is drilled centrally through one face of the cube at right angles to the larger holes.

Part D — Hinge Bar is a 120 mm ($4\frac{3}{4}$ in.) length of 9 mm ($\frac{3}{8}$ in.) diameter dowelling, which forms the pivot linking the Platform, via the Bearings, to the Uprights — Parts F.

Part E — Crosspiece is a simple rectangle with slots cut into its upper edge, to hold the two Uprights — Parts F — in position.

Parts F — Uprights are parallel vertical members, with slots cut into their lower edges matched to those in the Crosspiece, to which they are eventually glued. Each Upright has a hole drilled through it to freely accept the 9 mm ($\frac{3}{8}$ in.) diameter Hinge Bar, so that it can rotate easily. The Uprights and Crosspiece together bear the weight of the Platform and teapot, also providing a stable base upon which the latter can be pivoted.

Parts G — Fences are securely slotted into the Platform — Part A — at right angles to it and to each other, leaving a slot between the Fences, through which the teapot spout protrudes. The Fences hold the teapot in place whilst it is tilted for pouring.

Assembly

1 Pin and glue the Handle — Part B — to the rear underside of the Platform — Part A. Hereafter the entire unit may be assembled without glueing.

2 Enter the two screws through the holes in the front of the Platform — Part A — and into the pilot holes in the Bearings — Parts C — so as to hold the

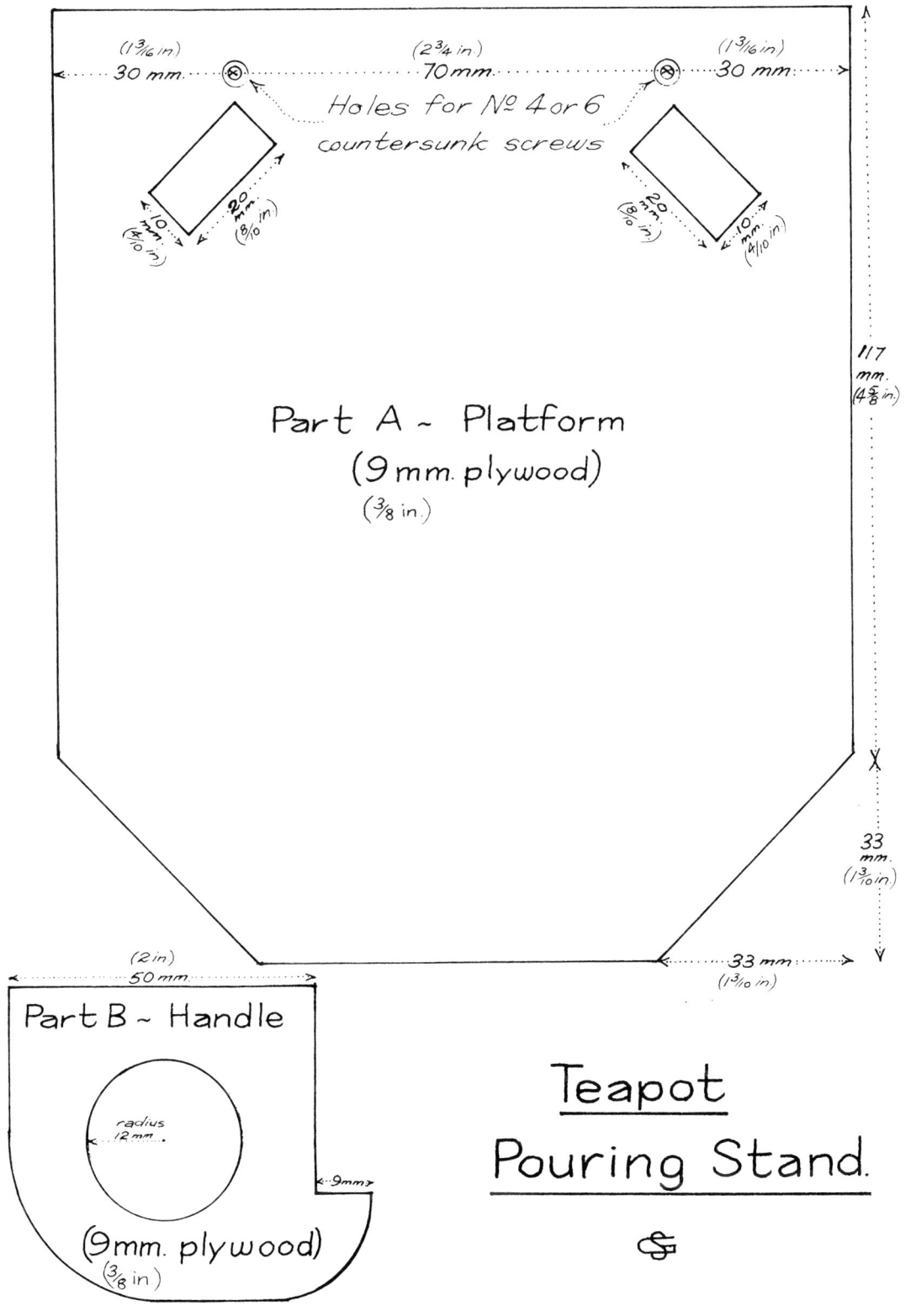

(1 3/16 in.)
30 mm.

(2 3/4 in.)
70mm.

(1 3/16 in.)
30 mm.

Holes for № 4 or 6
countersunk screws

20
mm
(8/10 in.)

10
mm
(4/10 in.)

20
mm
(8/10 in.)

10
mm
(4/10 in.)

Part A ~ Platform
(9 mm. plywood)
(3/8 in.)

117
mm.
(4 5/8 in.)

33
mm.
(1 3/10 in.)

33 mm
(1 3/10 in.)

(2 in.)
50 mm.

Part B ~ Handle

radius
12 mm.

9mm

(9mm. plywood)
(3/8 in.)

Teapot
Pouring Stand.

GS

75

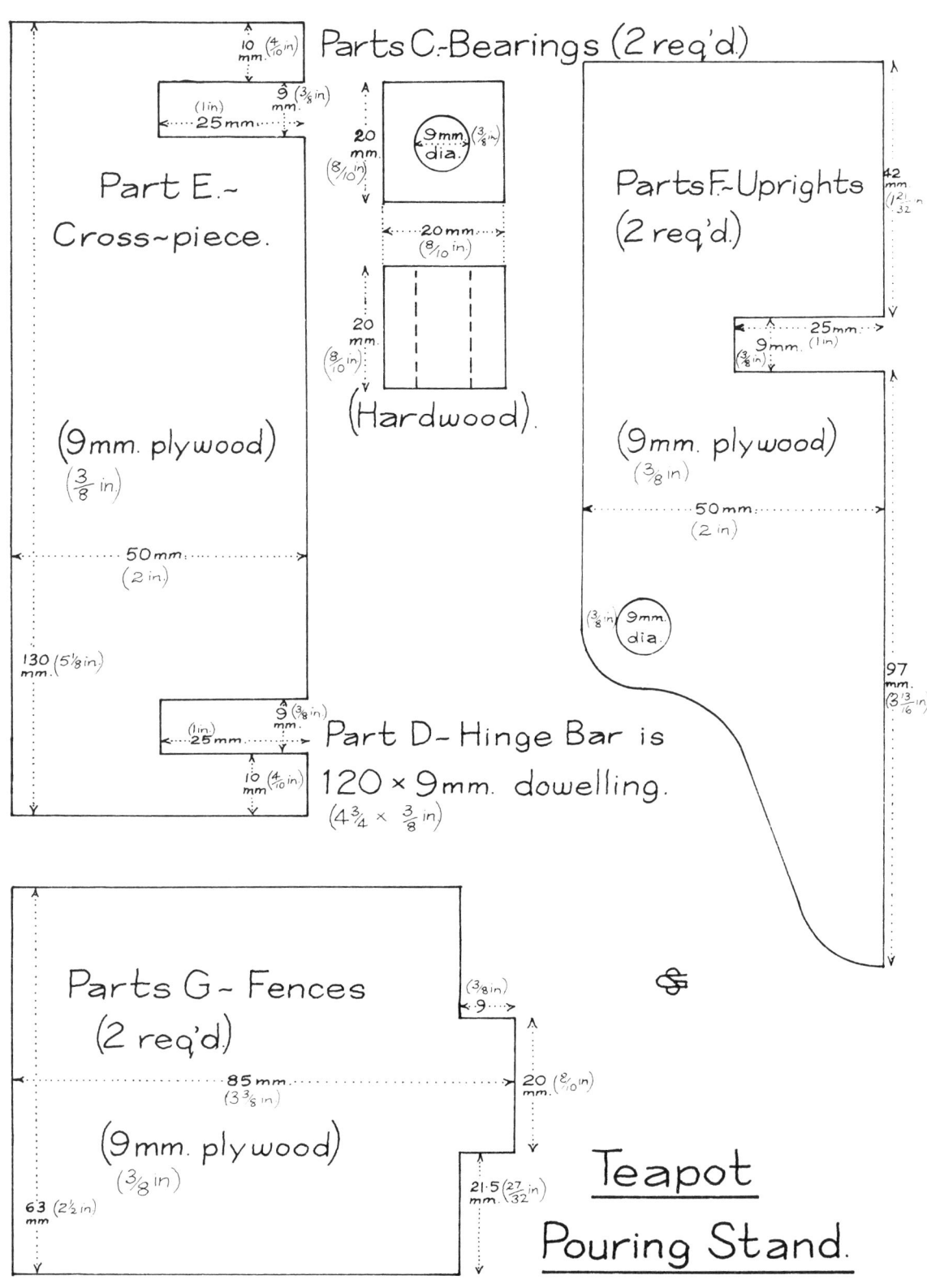

Parts C-Bearings (2 req'd.)

10 mm (⁴/₁₀ in)

(1 in) 25mm

9 mm (³/₈ in)

Part E.– Cross-piece.

(9mm. plywood) (³/₈ in.)

50mm (2 in)

130 mm (5⅛ in.)

(1 in) 25mm

9 mm (³/₈ in.)

10 mm (⁴/₁₀ in)

20 mm (⁸/₁₀ in)

9mm (³/₈ in) dia.

20mm (⁸/₁₀ in)

20 mm (⁸/₁₀ in)

(Hardwood).

Part D– Hinge Bar is 120 × 9mm. dowelling. (4¾ × ³/₈ in)

Parts F.-Uprights (2 req'd.)

42 mm (1²¹/₃₂ in)

25mm 9mm (1 in) (³/₈ in)

(9mm. plywood) (³/₈ in.)

50mm (2 in)

(³/₈ in) 9mm. dia.

97 mm (3¹³/₁₆ in)

Parts G – Fences (2 req'd.)

(³/₈ in) ⸱9⸱

85mm (3³/₈ in)

(9mm. plywood) (³/₈ In)

63 mm (2½ in)

20 mm (⁸/₁₀ in)

21·5 mm (²⁷/₃₂ in)

Teapot Pouring Stand.

76

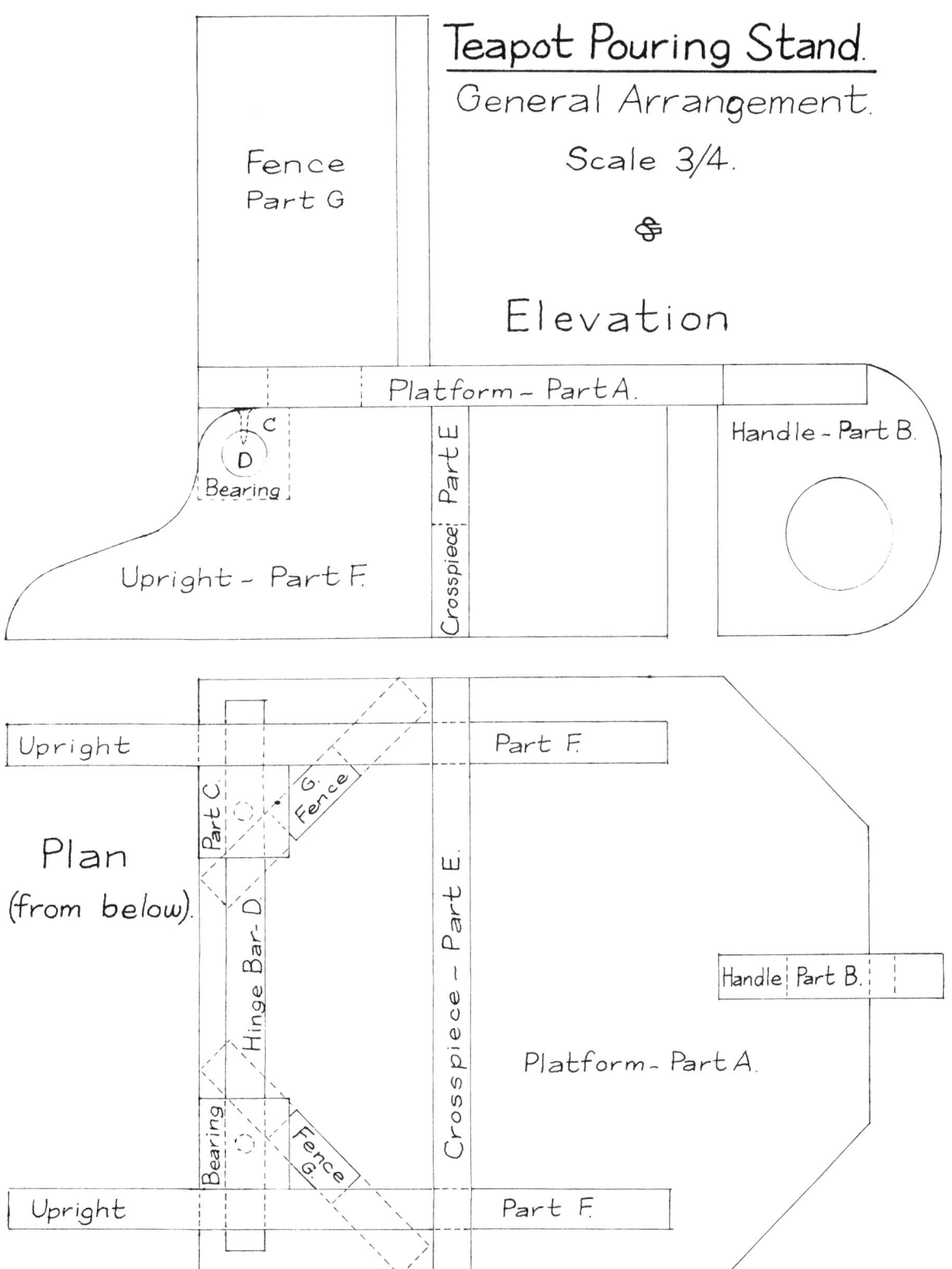

Teapot Pouring Stand.
General Arrangement.
Scale 3/4.

Elevation

Fence
Part G

Platform – Part A.

C
D
Bearing

Handle – Part B.

Crosspiece – Part E

Upright – Part F.

Plan
(from below).

Upright

Part F.

Part C.

G.
Fence

Hinge Bar – D

Crosspiece – Part E.

Handle ¦ Part B.

Bearing

Fence
G.

Platform – Part A.

Upright

Part F.

latter in position but leave clear the 9 mm ($\frac{3}{8}$ in.) holes.

3 Position the Hinge Bar — Part D — through the holes in the Bearings — Parts C — so that is protrudes an equal amount at each end, then secure it in place by completely driving home the two screws holding the Bearings — Parts C — to the Platform — Part A.

4 Each protruding end of the Hinge Bar — Part D — now should be passed through the hole in one of the Uprights — Parts F.

5 Secure the two Uprights in position by push-fitting their slots into the matching slots in the Crosspiece — Part E.

6 Place the two Fences — Parts G — in their slots at the front of the Platform.

By raising the Handle it should be possible now to tilt the Platform easily which should be secure enough to try out teapots for size and suitability; but, to be on the safe side, use only cold water at

Finishing

After sanding down the surfaces, a suitable wood sealer should be applied and, when that is dry, either paint or varnish. It is a good idea to glue a circular table mat of about 120 mm ($4\frac{3}{4}$ in.) dia. made from cork or similar non-slip material onto the top of the platform to protect it from the heat of the teapot in use.

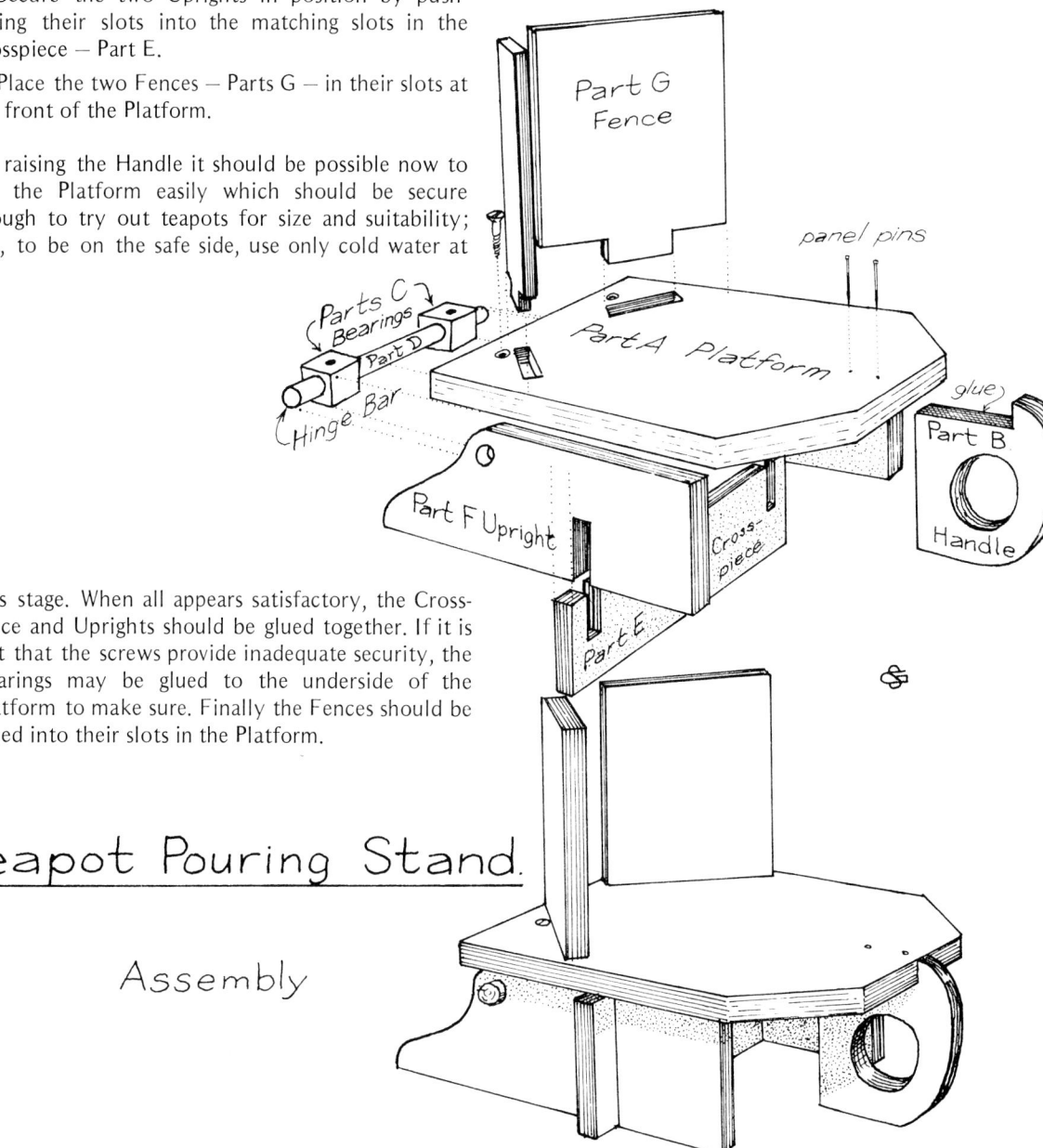

this stage. When all appears satisfactory, the Crosspiece and Uprights should be glued together. If it is felt that the screws provide inadequate security, the Bearings may be glued to the underside of the Platform to make sure. Finally the Fences should be glued into their slots in the Platform.

Teapot Pouring Stand.

Assembly

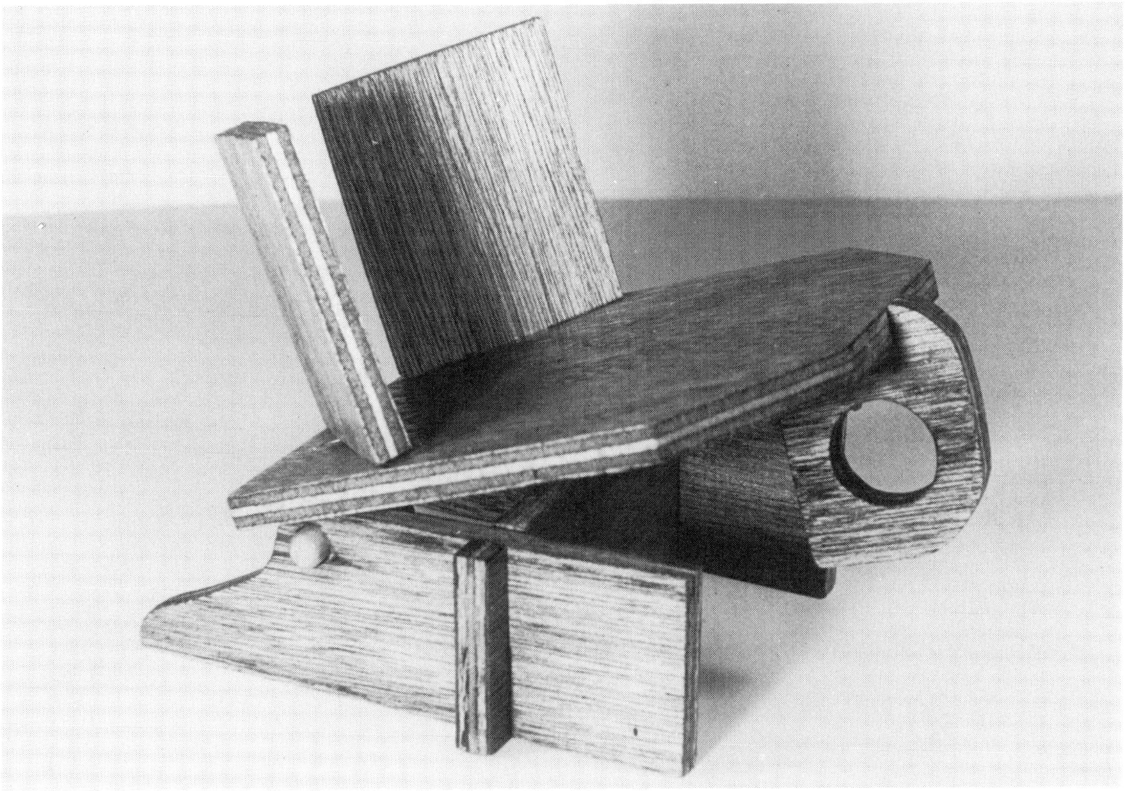

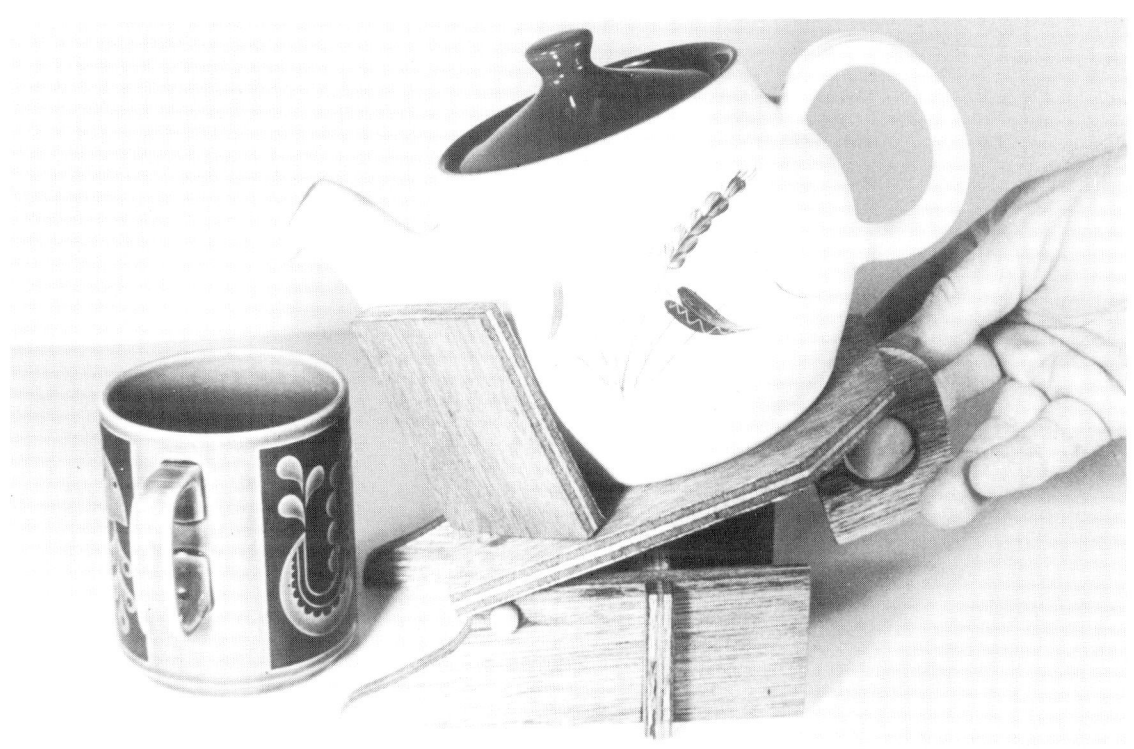

Pouring Stand tilted to show construction

Pouring Stand with teapot and mug

FOLDING BED TABLE

This might be described as the traditional design of Folding Bed Table, the purpose of which is to provide a stable platform across, but clear of, the body of a person lying or sitting in bed, so that meals may be served, jigsaw puzzles solved, patience cards manipulated and letters written with the maximum convenience. When no longer required, the Bed Table's legs can be folded underneath its top, to store away in the minimum of space until it is needed again.

Components

Part A – Top A rectangle of 9 mm ($\frac{3}{8}$ in.) plywood 350 x 550 mm ($13\frac{3}{4}$ x $21\frac{3}{4}$ in.) with the corners rounded off to a radius of about 20 mm ($\frac{3}{4}$ in.).

Part B – Legs Two of these Parts are required, being cut, together with the two Parts F – Latches – most economically from a rectangle of 9 mm ($\frac{3}{8}$ in.) plywood 400 x 245 mm ($15\frac{3}{4}$ x $9\frac{5}{8}$ in.) in accordance with the layout provided on page 82.

Part C – Centre This is a simple square 100 x 100 mm (4 x 4 in.) of wood 25 mm (1 in.) thick. The type of wood used is not important, as long as it provides good holding for screws.

Part D – Spring A simple rectangle of 4 mm ($\frac{3}{16}$ in.) plywood 550 x 100 mm ($21\frac{5}{8}$ x 4 in.). This should be cut so that the grain in the majority of the layers of the plywood runs lengthwise, so that the firmest spring is provided.

Parts E – Leg Stops These are not absolutely essential, but are recommended as they relieve stress on the Hinges, which may eventually work loose if Leg Stops are not fitted. They are made from two 300 mm ($11\frac{13}{16}$ in.) lengths of 20 mm ($\frac{3}{4}$ in.) square section hardwood.

Parts F – Latches These two parts hold the Legs upright on the inner side, against the Spring. As mentioned under Parts B above, Parts F are cut, together with Parts B, from a rectangle of 9 mm ($\frac{3}{8}$ in.) plywood. Each Latch is a rectangle 100 x 45 mm ($3\frac{15}{16}$ x $1\frac{3}{4}$ in.).

Fiddles These are fitted along the sides and ends of the Top, with a gap at the corners, projecting 9 mm ($\frac{3}{8}$ in.) above the level of the Table, so as to prevent objects sliding off if the Table is tilted inadvertently. The gaps at the corners are left to facilitate brushing off crumbs and wiping clean. The side Fiddles are 500 mm ($19\frac{11}{16}$ in.) long and the end Fiddles 320 mm ($12\frac{5}{8}$ in.) long, all being 18 mm ($\frac{3}{4}$ in.) wide and cut from 4 mm ($\frac{3}{16}$ in.) thick plywood. The projecting corners are rounded off.

Hinges Four of these are needed, preferably of brass and from 60 to 80 mm ($2\frac{3}{8}$ to $3\frac{1}{8}$ in.) long. They should be provided with suitable screws to hold in 9 mm ($\frac{3}{8}$ in.) plywood.

Screws Preferably brass, in addition to those needed for the Hinges; eight No. 8 x 12 mm ($\frac{1}{2}$ in.) countersunk, and ten No. 8 x 16 mm ($\frac{5}{8}$ in.) countersunk.

Pins and Glue Some 20 to 30 small panel pins and a little wood glue are needed to fix the Fiddles to the Top.

Assembly

1 Cut all Parts in accordance with the drawings and specifications, and give all surfaces a smooth finish with glasspaper.

2 Drill holes for screws where indicated and countersink as necessary.

3 Glue and pin Fiddles to the sides and ends of Part A – Top.

4 Screw Part A – Top – and Part C – Centre – together with four No. 8 x 16 mm ($\frac{5}{8}$ in.) screws entered from above.

5 Screw the Hinges to Parts B – Legs – in the positions indicated.

6 Screw Parts E – Leg Stops – and Part A – Top – together, with six No. 8 x 16 mm ($\frac{5}{8}$ in.) screws (three per Part E), entered from above.

7 Fix each Part B – Legs – in position on Part A – Top – hard up against each Part E – Leg Stop – by screwing the Hinges to Part A – Top – and test to ensure that they fold flat.

8 Fix Part D – Spring – in position on Part C – Centre – with four No. 8 x 12 mm ($\frac{1}{2}$ in.) screws, entered from below.

9 Fix Parts F – Latches – in position on Part D – Spring – so that they are hard up against their respective Parts B – Legs – which they hold upright, with four No. 8 x 12 mm ($\frac{1}{2}$ in.) screws (two per Latch). Test to ensure that the Latches operate smoothly and securely, locking the Legs as they unfold into the upright position.

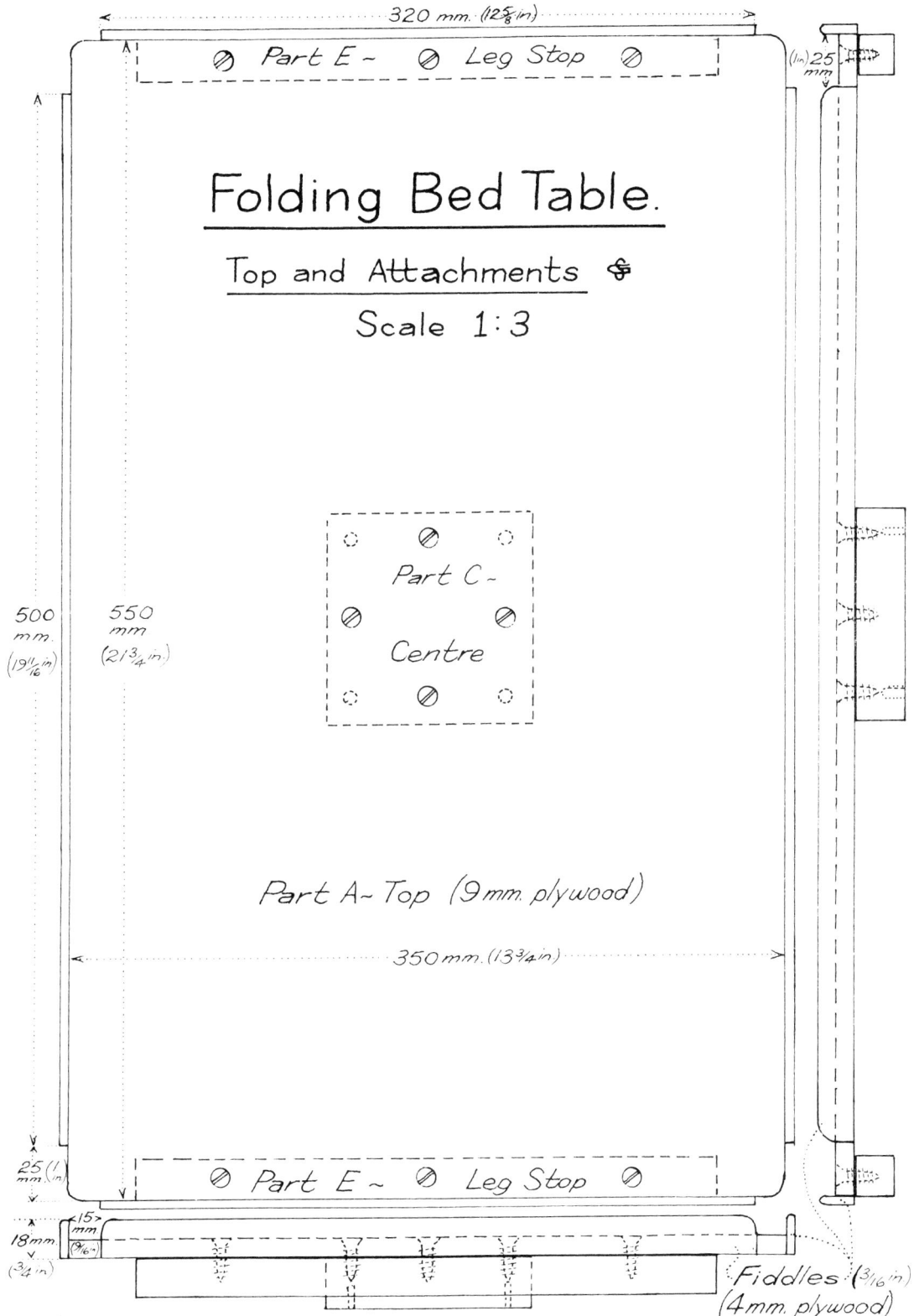

320 mm. (12⅝in)

Part E ~ Leg Stop

(1in) 25 mm

Folding Bed Table.

Top and Attachments ⚬

Scale 1:3

Part C ~

Centre

500 mm. (19¹¹⁄₁₆in)

550 mm (21¾in.)

Part A~ Top (9mm. plywood)

350 mm. (13¾in)

Part E ~ Leg Stop

25 (1 mm in)

15 mm (9⁄16")

18mm (¾in)

Fiddles (³⁄₁₆in) (4mm. plywood)

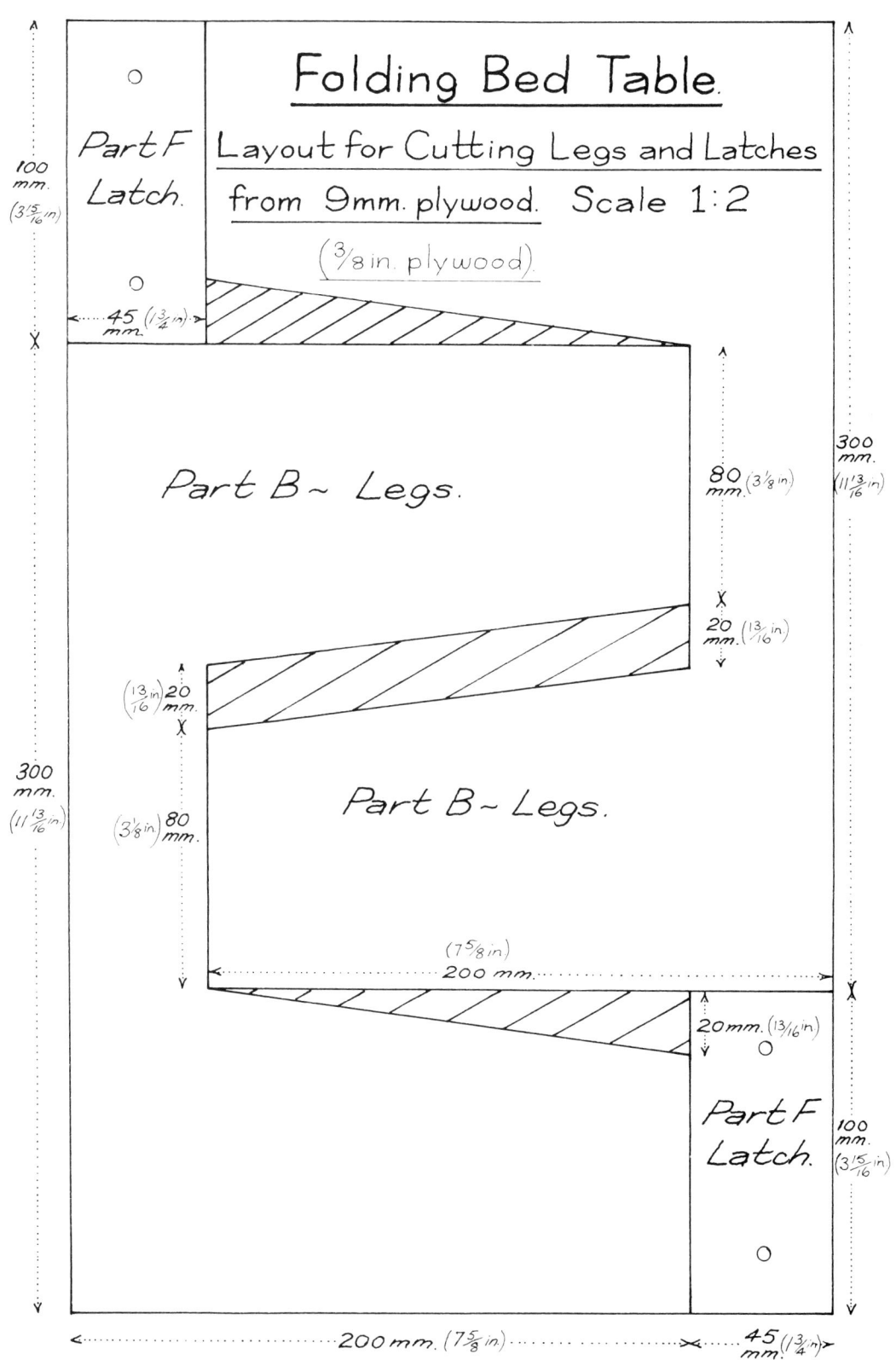

Folding Bed Table.

Layout for Cutting Legs and Latches from 9mm. plywood. Scale 1:2

$(^3/_8$ in. plywood$)$

Part F
Latch.

Part B ~ Legs.

Part B ~ Legs.

Part F
Latch.

100 mm. $(3^5/_{16}$in$)$

45 mm $(1^3/_4$in$)$

300 mm. $(11^{13}/_{16}$in$)$

80 mm. $(3^1/_8$in$)$

20 mm. $(13/_{16}$in$)$

$(13/_{16}$in$)$ 20 mm.

$(3^1/_8$in$)$ 80 mm.

$(7^5/_8$in$)$
200 mm.

300 mm. $(11^{13}/_{16}$in$)$

20mm. $(13/_{16}$in$)$

100 mm. $(3^{15}/_{16}$in$)$

200 mm. $(7^5/_8$in$)$

45 mm. $(1^3/_4$in$)$

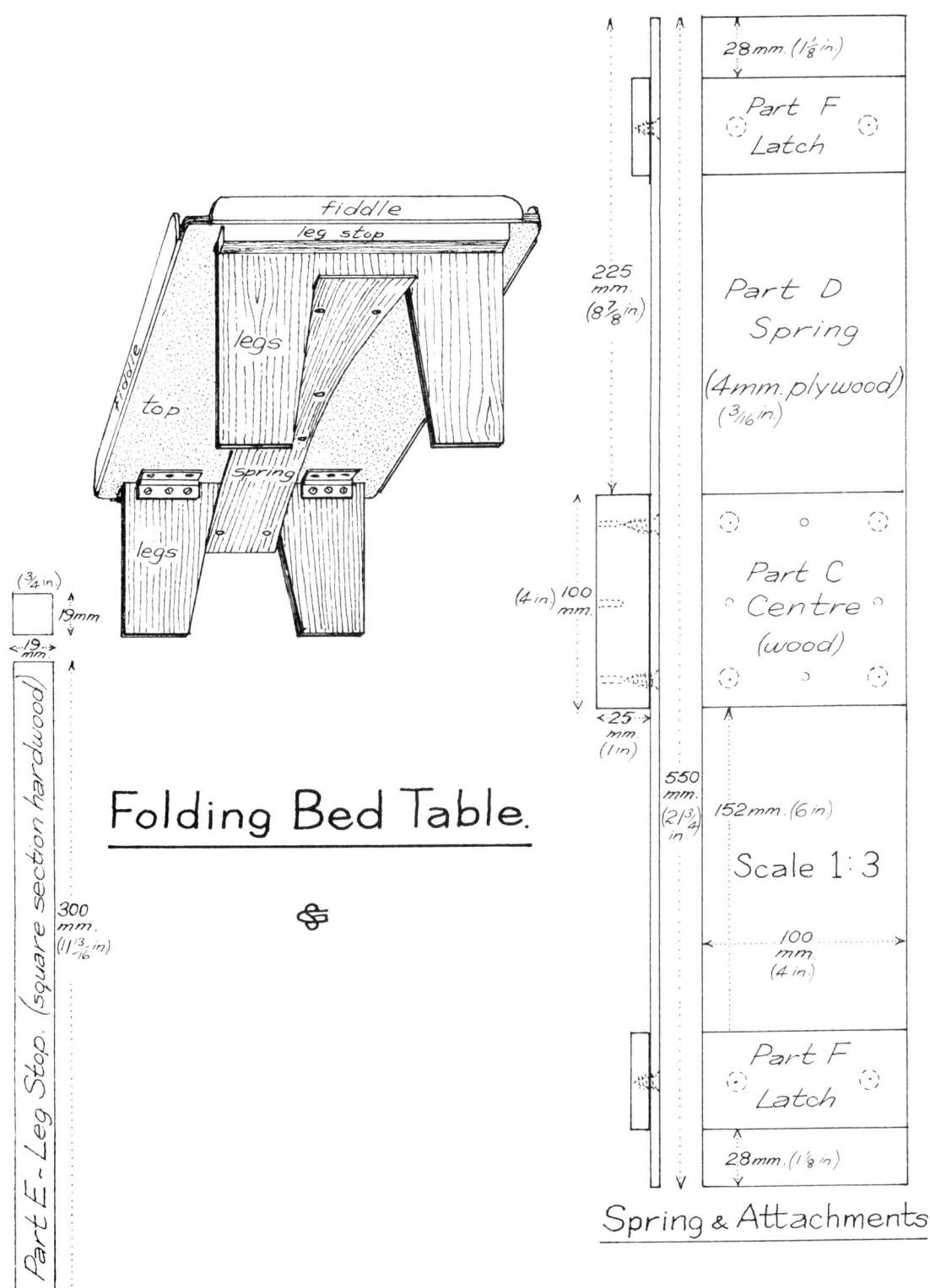

fiddle

leg stop

legs

top

fiddle

spring

legs

Folding Bed Table.

(¾ in)

19mm

19 mm.

300 mm. (11³⁄₁₆ in)

Part E ~ Leg Stop. (square section hardwood)

28mm. (1⅛ in)

Part F
Latch

225 mm. (8⅞ in)

Part D
Spring
(4mm. plywood)
(³⁄₁₆ in.)

(4 in) 100 mm.

Part C
Centre
(wood)

25 mm. (1 in)

550 mm. (21¾ in)

152mm. (6 in.)

Scale 1:3

100 mm. (4 in.)

Part F
Latch

28mm. (1⅛ in)

Spring & Attachments

Folding
Bed Table.

General Arrangement.
Scale 1:4

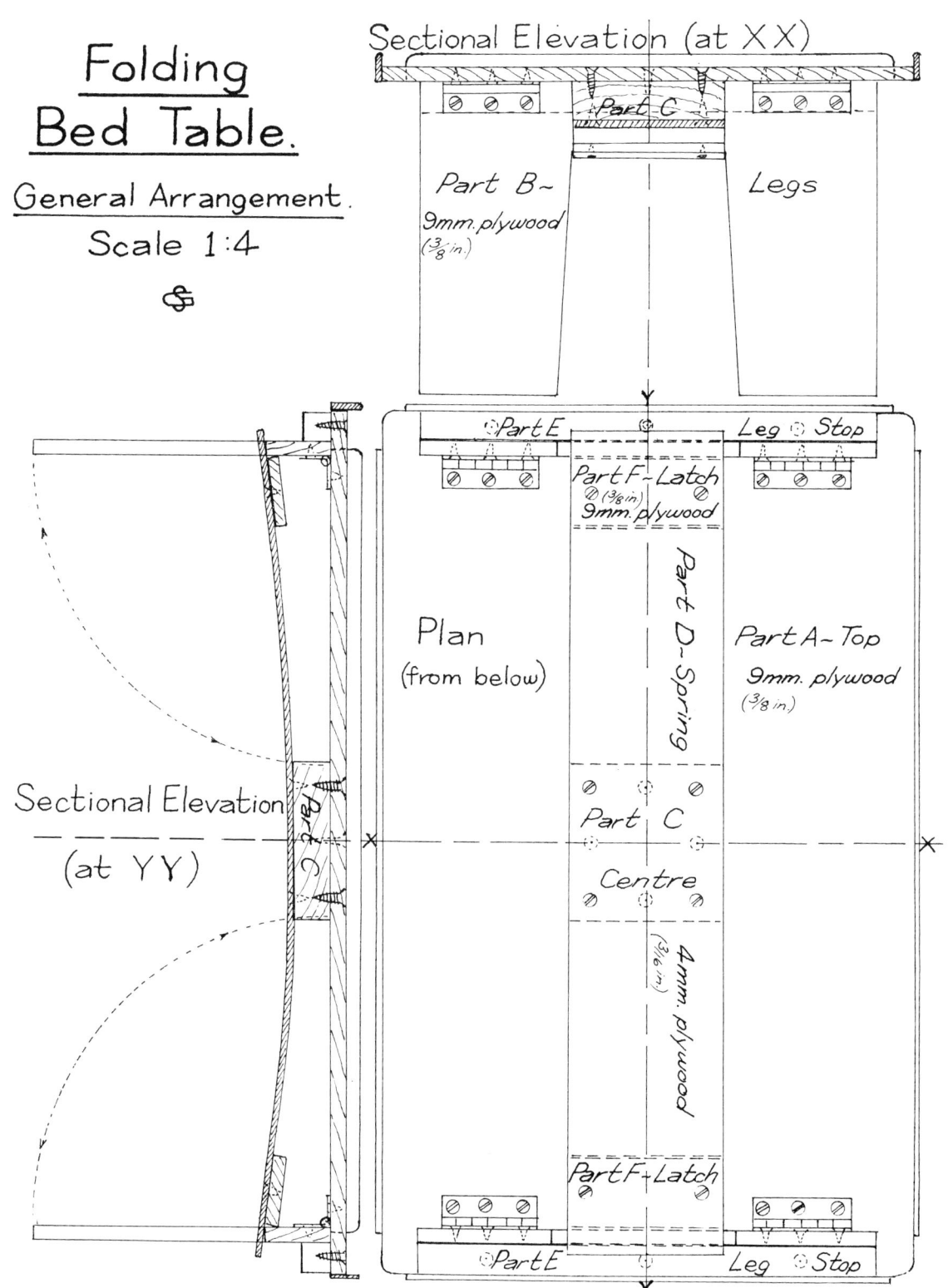

Sectional Elevation (at XX)

Part B~
9mm. plywood
($\frac{3}{8}$ in.)

Part C

Legs

Sectional Elevation

(at YY)

Part C

Plan
(from below)

Part E

Leg ⊙ Stop

Part F~Latch
(⊘ ($\frac{3}{8}$ in.)
9mm. plywood

Part A~ Top
9mm. plywood
($\frac{3}{8}$ in.)

Part D~Spring

Part C

Centre

4mm. plywood
($\frac{3}{16}$ in.)

Part F~Latch

Part E

Leg ⊙ Stop

84

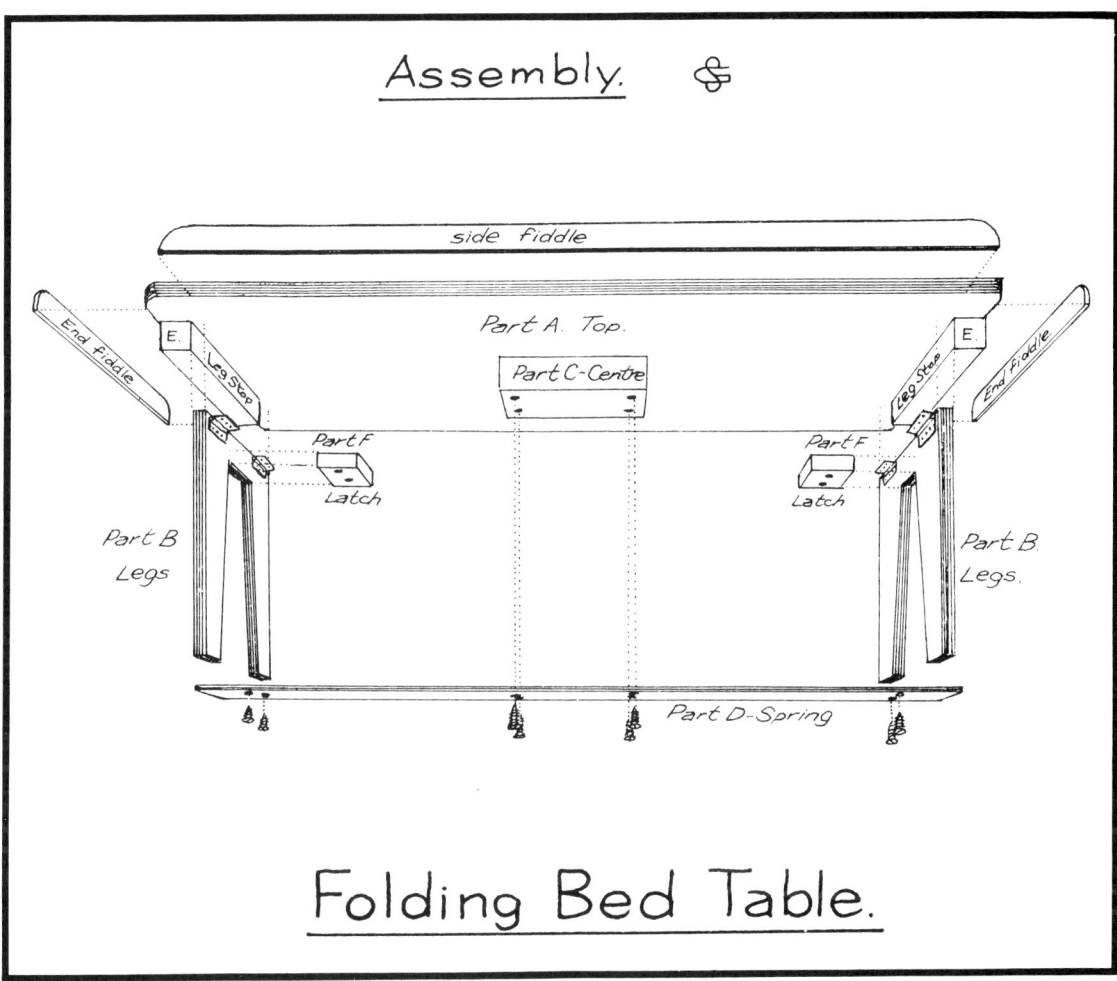

Assembly.

side fiddle

End Fiddle

E.

Leg Stop

Part A. Top.

Part C-Centre

Part F

Latch

Part B
Legs

E.

Leg Stop

End Fiddle

Part F

Latch

Part B.
Legs.

Part D-Spring

Folding Bed Table.

Finishing

The Folding Bed Table is an item which, if properly made, could easily outlast several generations, so it is worth finishing it well to ensure that it can be kept clean. The upper surface of the Top can be covered with a self-adhesive plastic film, such as Fablon or, better still, with a hardwearing plastic laminated sheet, such as Formica, which has to be glued into place with a contact adhesive. The remaining surfaces, after being carefully smoothed down with glasspaper, should be sealed with a suitable wood sealer and then given at least two coats of undercoat and one of gloss paint or, if varnish is preferred, not less than three coats of varnish, rubbing down lightly with glasspaper after the first and second coats.

Storing

The Folding Bed Table can be stored in very little space, at the back of a cupboard or on top of a wardrobe for instance, but before putting it away for any appreciable length of time it is worth placing a drop of light oil on each Hinge and then sliding the whole Table into a polythene bag of a suitable size, the type of bag used to line swing-bins being ideal. This will ensure that, on the next occasion when you have an invalid in bed, the Bed Table is clean and ready for immediate use. (See page 86 for photographs of the finished table.)

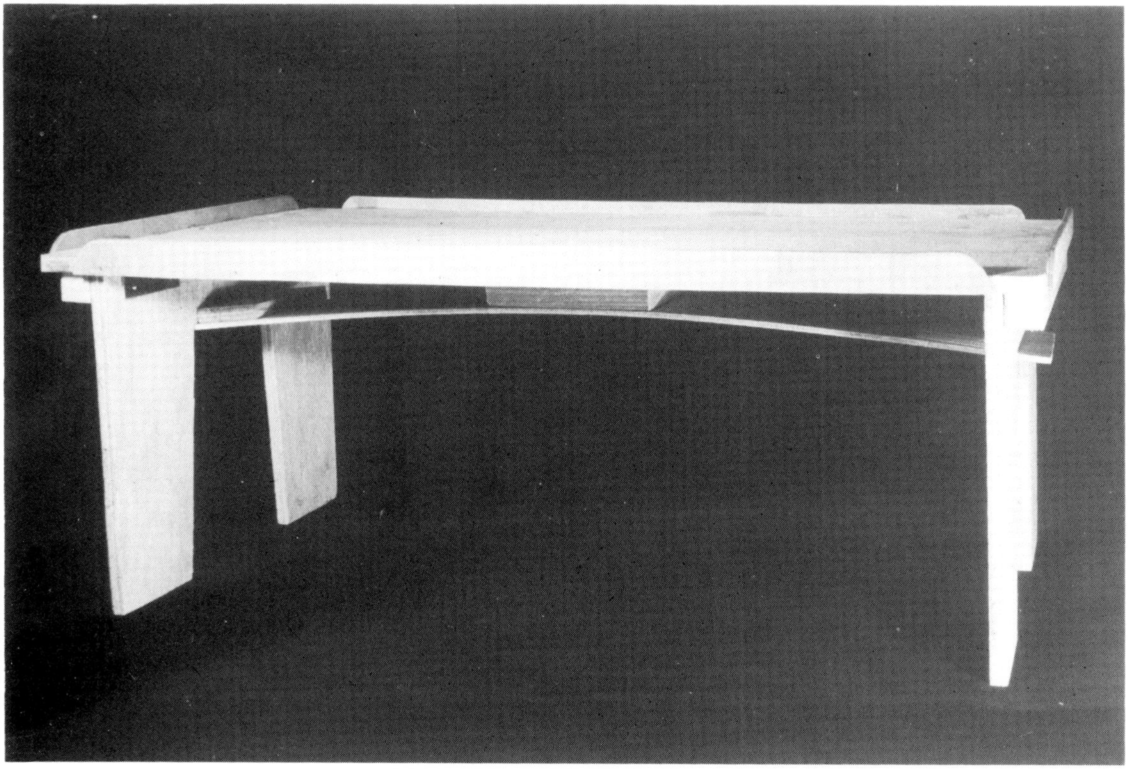

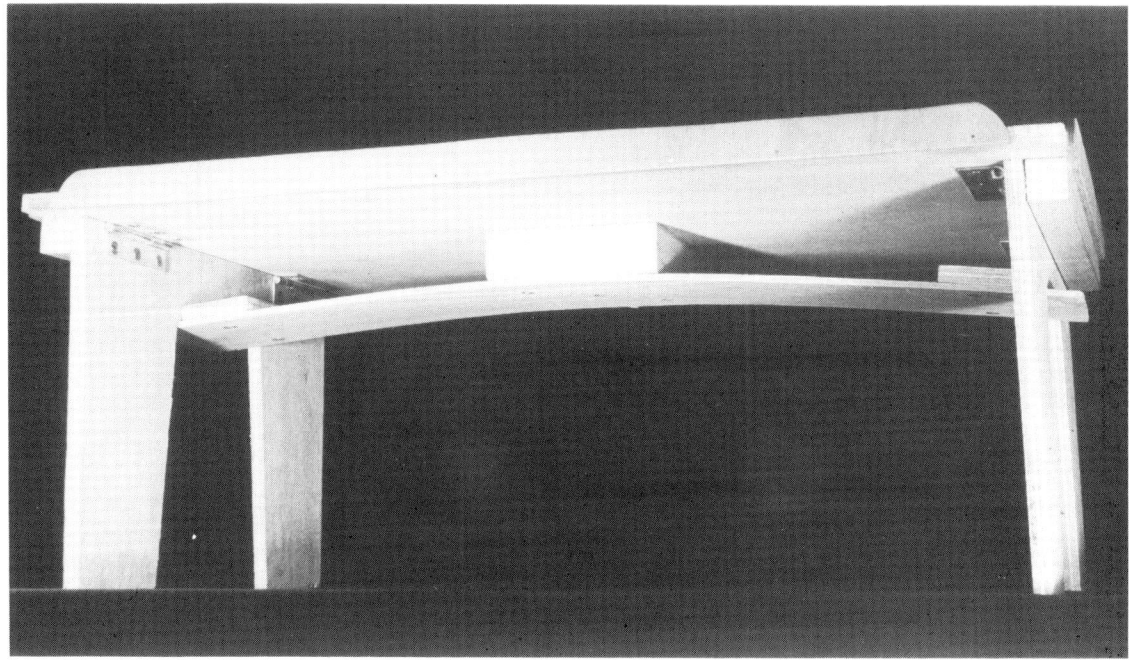

Folding Bed Table assembled ready for sealing
and painting or varnishing — side view

Folding Bed Table — view from underneath

PLAYING CARD HOLDER

Card games, such as bridge, whist and rummy, to name only three, are very popular, particularly among the older members of the community, but people with arthritic hands, or with the use of only one hand, can find it very difficult to hold a hand of cards for any length of time, if at all. This device, which is simplicity itself, provides a means of holding a hand of playing cards vertically on a table, so that they can not be seen by other players and can be easily picked up and replaced.

The Playing Card Holder as illustrated was made from a rectangular block of mahogany, $7\frac{1}{2}$ inches long, $\frac{3}{4}$ inch high and $1\frac{3}{4}$ inches wide (190 mm x 19 mm x 44 mm), but these dimensions are in no way critical and almost any kind of wood will do,

although a hardwood is probably best, because, being dense, it tends to be heavier and therefore more stable for this purpose than softwoods. The slots were sawn vertically, half an inch (12 mm) apart, using a fine-toothed tenon saw, to approximately halfway through the block, at an angle of 45° to the sides. A hacksaw or junior hacksaw would do the job as well, but the slots should not be too wide, or the cards will loll at an angle instead of being held upright. The Holder illustrated has been french polished, for a truly up-market appearance, but such refinement is not really necessary. There are ten slots, which would be enough for most card games, particularly as each slot will hold more than one card if required.

The Playing Card Holder in use.

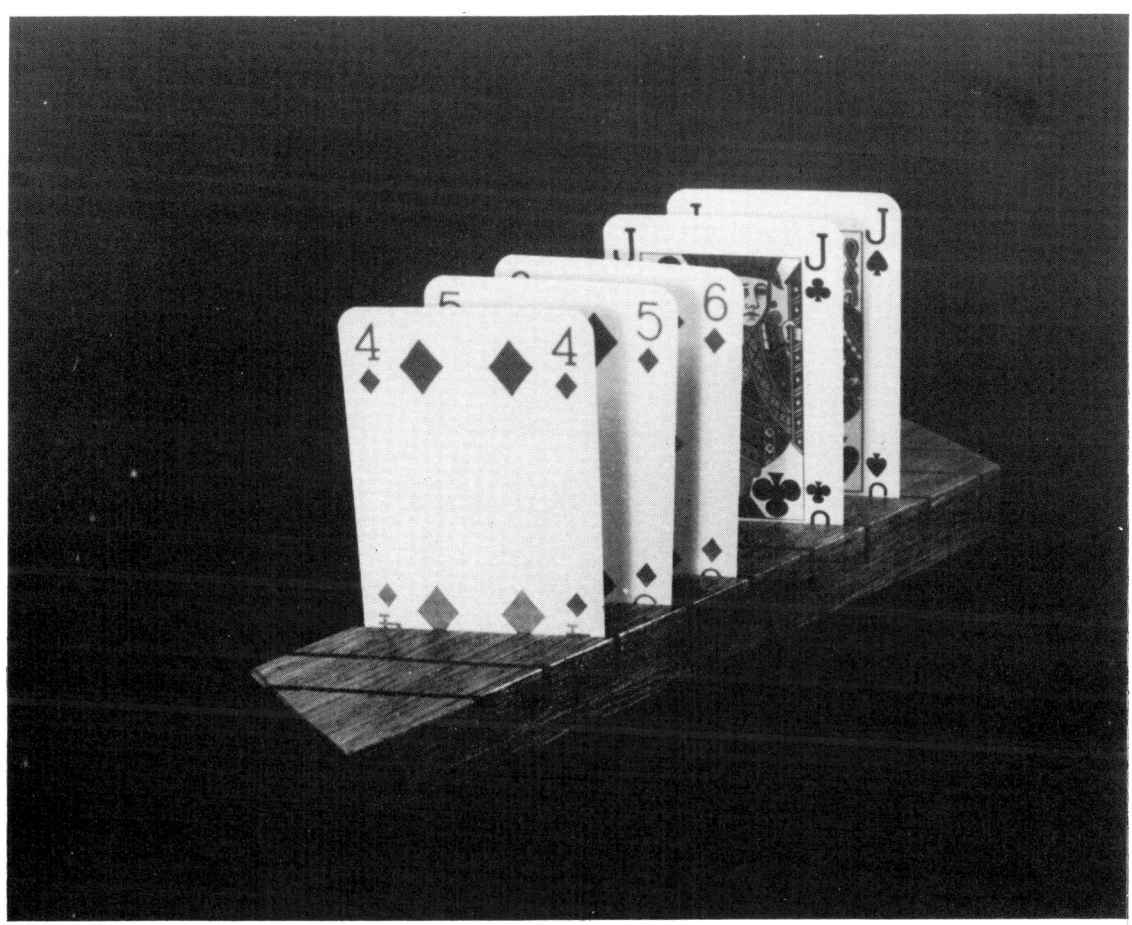

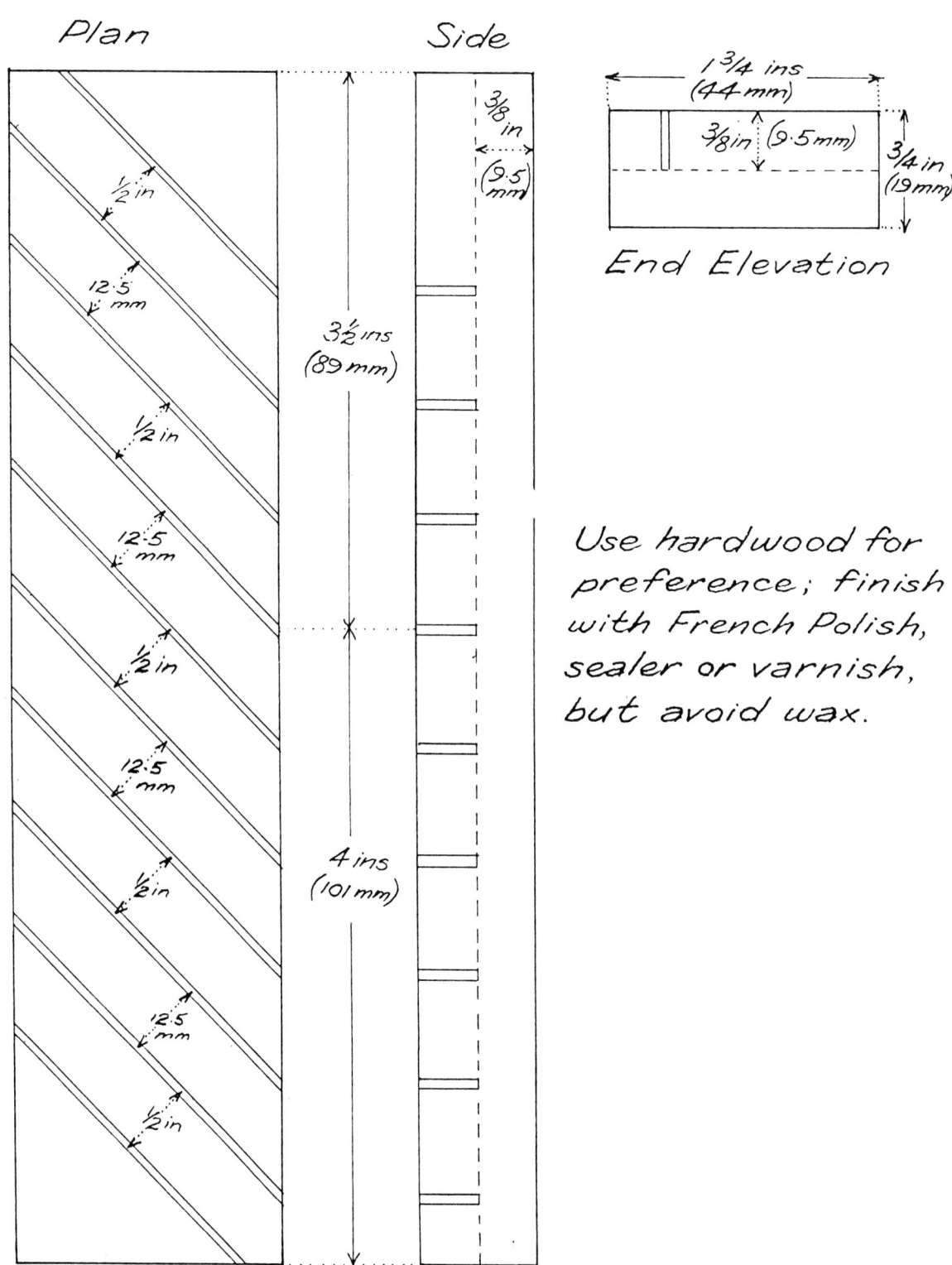

Plan

Side

½ in

12·5 mm

½ in

12·5 mm

½ in

12·5 mm

½ in

12·5 mm

½ in

12·5 mm

½ in

3⁸ in (9·5 mm)

3½ ins (89 mm)

4 ins (101 mm)

1³⁄₄ ins (44 mm)

3⁄8 in (9·5mm)

3⁄4 in (19 mm)

End Elevation

Use hardwood for preference; finish with French Polish, sealer or varnish, but avoid wax.

PLAYING CARD HOLDER.

LONG TROWEL & BULB PLANTER

In recent years, many new devices have become commercially available, which help to make gardening less physically arduous, and thus enable handicapped folk to pursue this popular and therapeutic hobby. In general, tools for gardening need to be industrially produced, because they require the strength of forged steel and welded joints. However, this tool does seem to fill a gap, in making it possible to place bulbs and corms precisely in position in the ground, without stooping or kneeling.

The tool is very simple, consisting of a short length of broom handle or dowelling screwed to about 3 feet (900 mm) of the type of plastic rainwater pipe sold for use on greenhouses and garden sheds. The plastic pipe is cut at an angle at both ends; at the lower end to provide a means of digging and filling holes in the soil and, at the upper end allowing the pipe to be screwed to the handle. About one third of the circumference of the handle

is flattened at its lower end to fit snugly against the pipe.

This tool can be used in any situation where a long-handled trowel may be useful, but it is not suitable for heavy digging, being primarily intended for planting bulbs, corms or large seeds, which can be dropped directly through the pipe into a prepared hole, furrow or trench, thus avoiding the need for bending, crouching or kneeling. The dimensions stated in the drawing were found convenient by the gentleman for whom the original tool was made. They may require adjustment for a particularly tall person, perhaps also for ladies and anyone in a wheelchair, but this is a simple matter of increasing or decreasing the length of one or both components slightly. If an increase is likely to be needed, make a generous allowance before any cutting is done. A reduction in length is easily made by cutting a little at a time from one end or from both, but once cut, it can not be stretched.

LONG TROWEL
AND BULB PLANTER

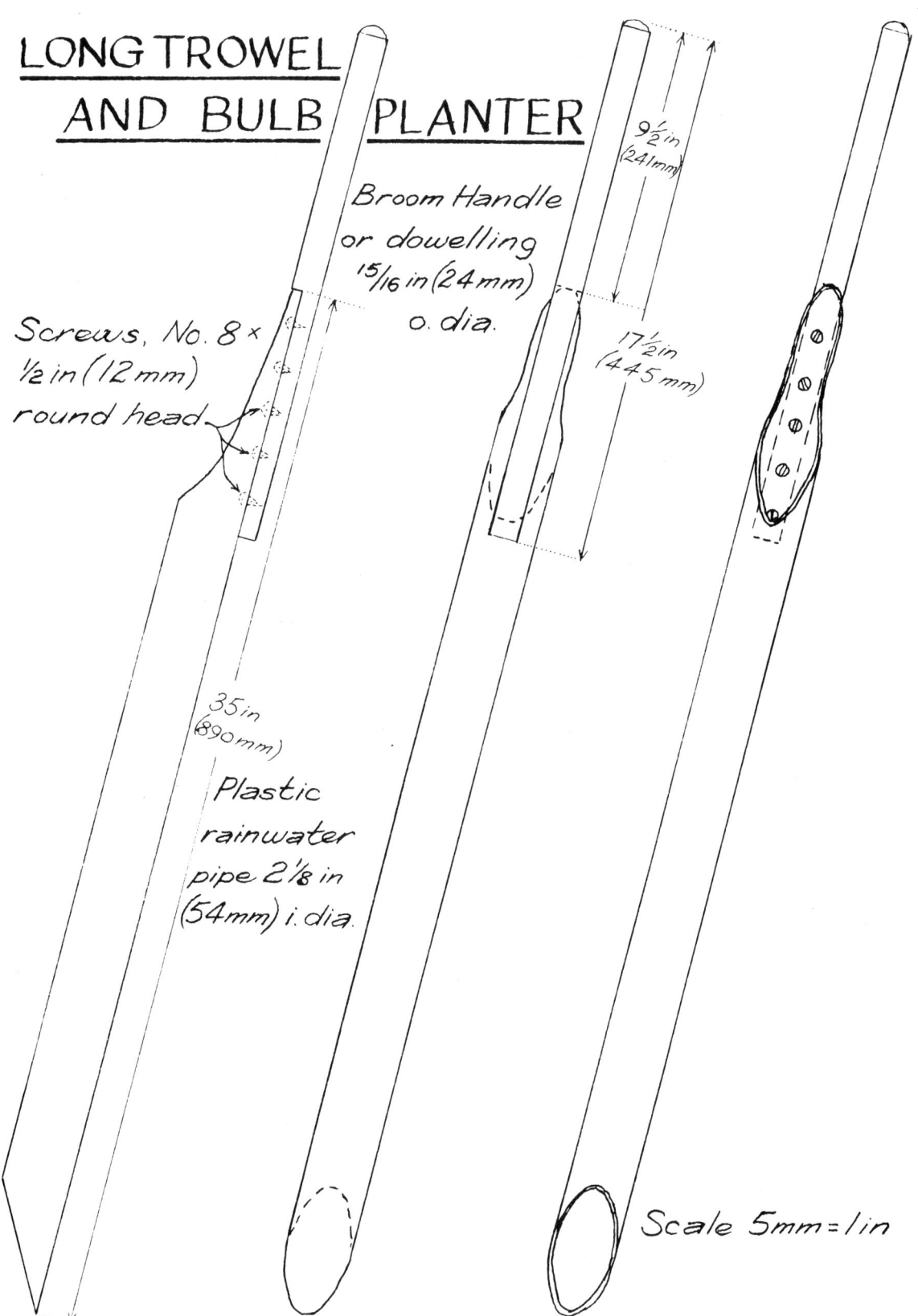

Broom Handle
or dowelling
$^{15}/_{16}$ in (24mm)
o. dia.

Screws, No. 8 ×
$^{1}/_{2}$ in (12 mm)
round head.

$9^{1}/_{2}$ in
(241mm)

$17^{1}/_{2}$ in
(445 mm)

35 in
(890 mm)

Plastic
rainwater
pipe $2^{1}/_{8}$ in
(54mm) i. dia.

Scale 5mm = 1in

SINGLE HAND KNIFE

This problem was raised by a gentleman who had lost an arm in World War II and found it difficult and occasionally embarrassing to eat away from home, because he could not cut some food into manageable morsels with only one hand. Normal table knives are designed for use in combination with a fork, which holds the item to be cut whilst the knife is used with a sawing motion. This needs two hands. Without the fork, the knife's sawing motion is ineffective and is liable to push items off the plate.

The requirement, therefore, was for a knife that would both cut and hold the object being cut at the same time. Experiment indicated that a half-moon shaped blade, with a horizontal handle along the top, such as cooks use for chopping in a turned hardwood bowl, would do the job, and so it proved. Such a knife is expensive, however, and not easy to make, really requiring special steel and cutting tools, so a simple way of producing a similar utensil was sought. The solution suggested here is simple and straightforward; a very cheap stainless steel soup spoon is modified in three basic steps, cutting off the lower part of the bowl, flattening the bowl and changing the shape of the handle.

A cheap spoon is better for the purpose, in that it is likely to be an uncomplicated shape and relatively easy to modify. Choose a spoon with as wide a bowl as can be found. Cut off the lower portion – about a third – with a hacksaw and then flatten the remainder of the bowl as much as possible, either by hammering it on a firm, flat surface, or by squeezing it between the jaws of a vice. In either method it is advisable to protect the stainless steel surface from scratching, otherwise you will have a lengthy polishing process to follow.

The cut edge should be filed to a smooth, shallow curve. This is the business part of the knife and care in its preparation is worthwhile. Forming the handle is just a matter of twisting the existing handle through a right angle and then rolling the end into a circular or oval shape. Any irregularities can be tapped out with a hammer over a simple former, such as a short length of dowel or broom handle. There is no obligation, of course, to form the handle as shown here; different users may favour different forms. It should be remembered, however, that the knife will need washing after use, so most kinds of wood are not recommended in forming a handle.

The design shown here has proved to be practical in use, unobtrusive and easily slipped into a plastic

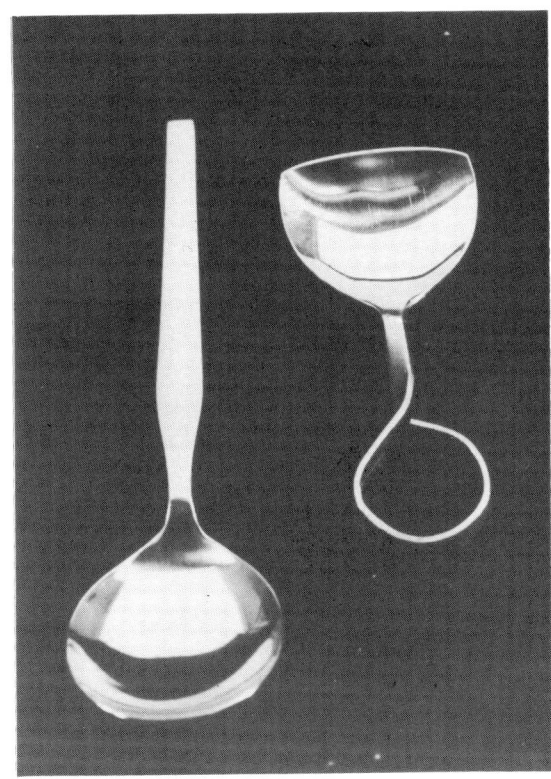

A Single Hand Knife alongside the type of soup spoon from which it was made.

bag for carrying in a pocket or purse. The knife should be kept sharp on a suitable stone and can be useful in the kitchen as well as at the dining table. It is important that the user remembers that it is a knife and is never tempted to use it as a spoon. This applies to all knives, of course, but since this one is derived from a spoon, a temptation to the absent-minded has to be acknowledged and guarded against. The cost is genuinely minimal, so the provision of two or three in different locations can be a reasonable proposition.

In use, the knife is placed vertically upon the item to be cut and is pressed downward. Instead of the sawing motion employed with conventional knives, this one is rocked to and fro along the cutting edge and will prove highly effective for most cutting and chopping purposes associated with food.

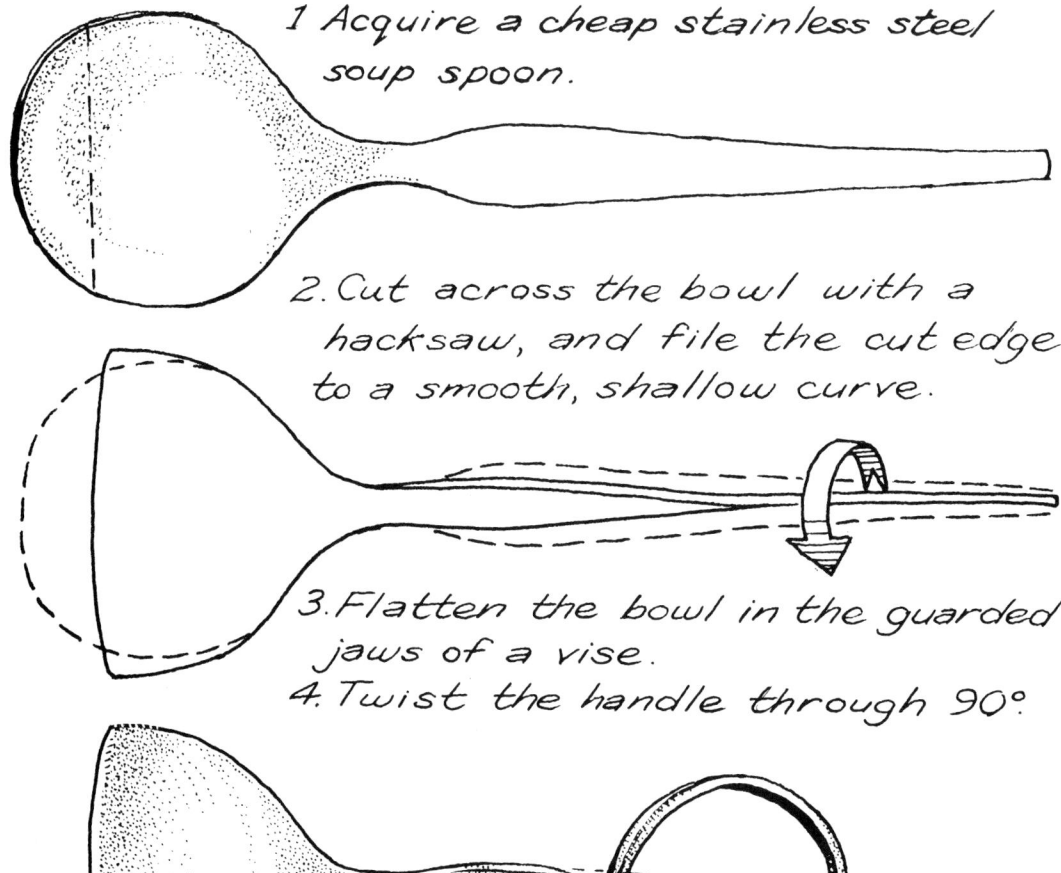

1 Acquire a cheap stainless steel soup spoon.

2. Cut across the bowl with a hacksaw, and file the cut edge to a smooth, shallow curve.

3. Flatten the bowl in the guarded jaws of a vise.

4. Twist the handle through 90°.

5. Hammer the handle into a circle around a rod or tube of suitable size & strength (e.g. broom handle) held in a vise.

6. Sharpen the cutting edge on a grindstone or oilstone to a keen smooth finish.

Single Hand Knife.

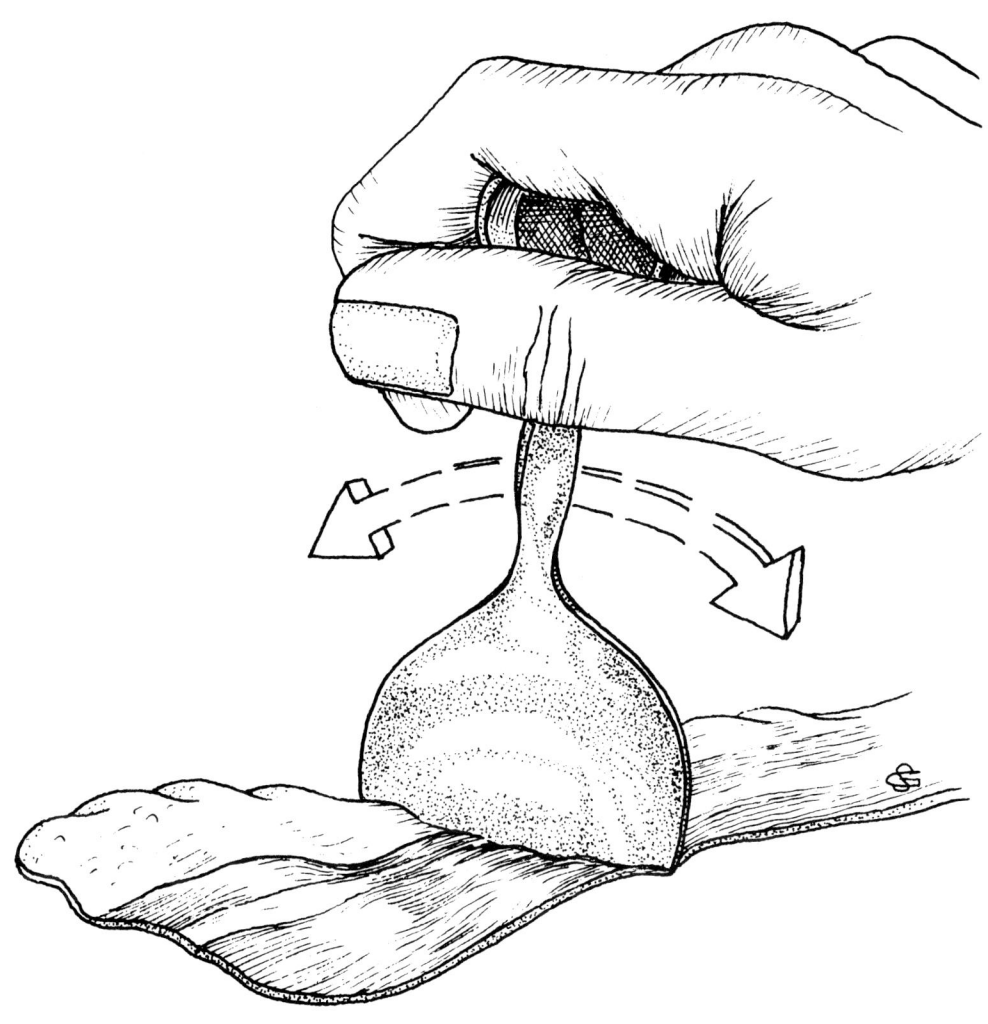

Cutting with the Single Hand Knife requires downward pressure combined with a rocking motion. Note that this utensil is intended for use as a knife, to cut with, not as a spoon or fork, for conveying food to the mouth. Use it in the American manner of using a table knife; cut first, then lay the knife aside and use a fork for eating the cut morsels. Do not risk a cut mouth!

BEDCLOTHES SUPPORT

A large number of people, many without disability, suffer some degree of discomfort from the weight and constriction of bedclothes on their feet, often causing cramp and circulation problems. This item is a simple, inexpensive and very easily constructed support, which allows the feet freedom of movement under the bedclothes. The support is clean and easily washable, but not cold or sharp to touch, and kind to sheets. It can be slipped into position when the occupant enters the bed and out again when the bed is not in use, and it can be dismantled or folded flat for storage in seconds.

Most large DIY stores and builders merchants stock a system of water overflow piping, having a standard internal diameter of about $\frac{3}{4}$ inch (19 mm) and made from white polypropylene or polyethylene. A range of fittings for joins and bends is usually available and this design uses two right angle bends and two T-joints. An important point to note is that none of the joints requires glue or solvents, as the fittings are designed with a taper providing a secure push-fit. This makes it possible to disassemble the unit for storage or transportation and to swing the 'feet' to align with the cross-piece, so the unit can lie flat for convenient daytime storage in a wardrobe or under the bed or divan. It is even light and convenient enough to tuck into an overnight bag.

The measurements provided here can be adjusted to suit the size of bed and the size of the occupant's feet, but are generally suitable for beds from 3 feet (915 mm) wide and upwards. Brands of such piping systems vary in the flexibility of the material used, so that it may be advisable to slide a piece of wooden dowelling of $\frac{3}{4}$ inch (19 mm) outside diameter, and approximately the same length as the crosspiece, inside the crosspiece, to prevent it from sagging under the weight of the bedclothes. The verticals and 'feet' should be quite rigid enough without such inserts.

If both occupants of a double bed wish to make use of a bedclothes support, one central vertical member with a T-joint at the top as well as the base, to link two crosspieces with the standard verticals at the sides, may provide a tidier unit than two separate ones.

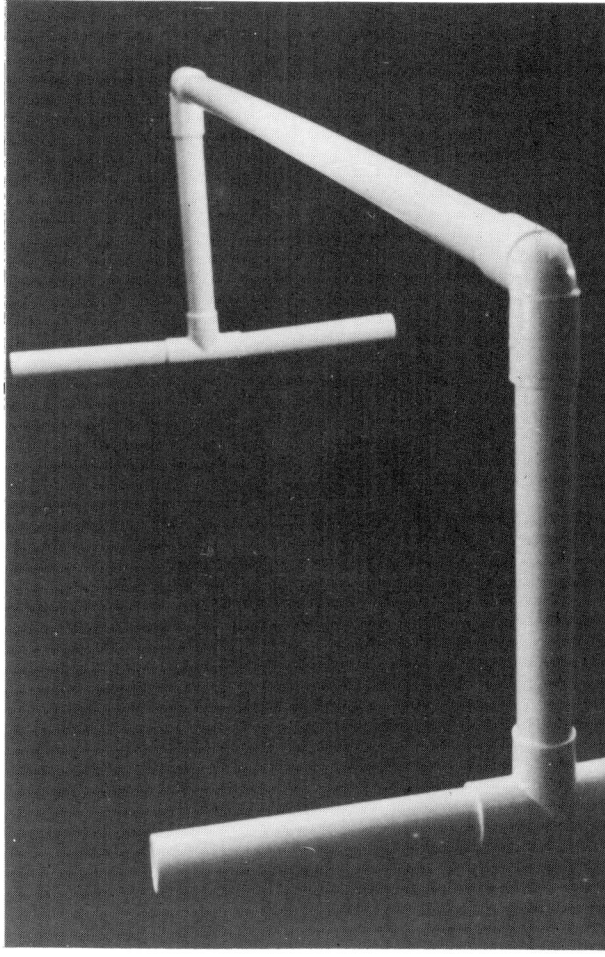

The Bedclothes Support assembled ready for use.

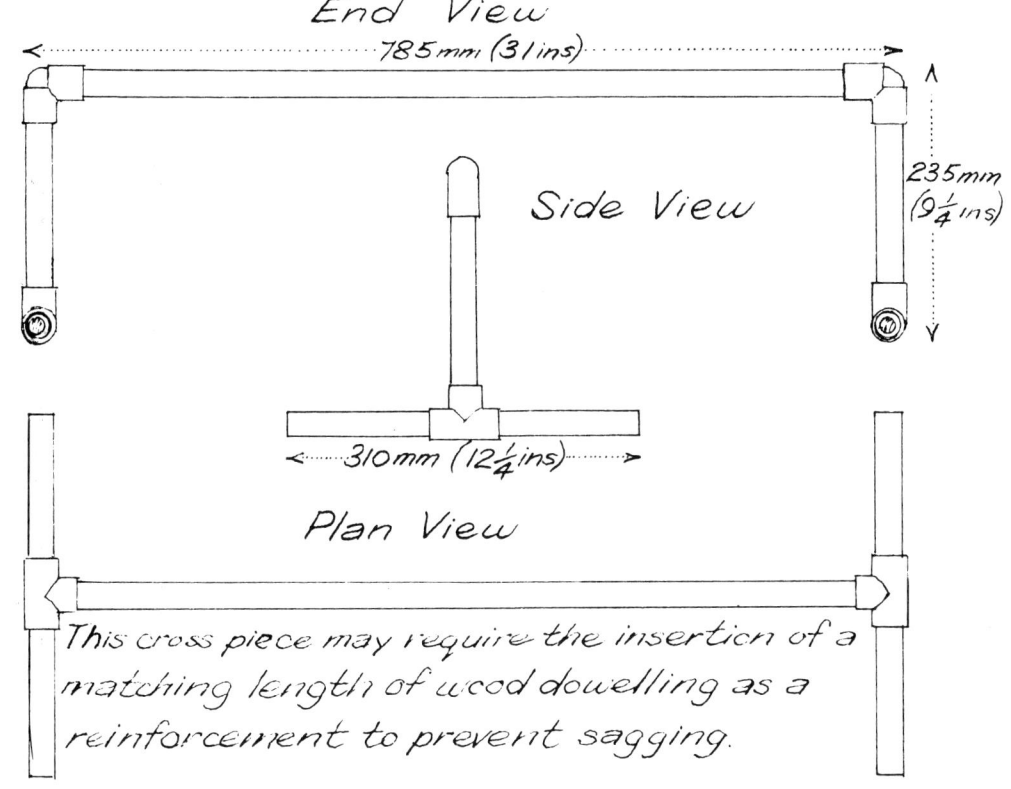

End View

785mm (31 ins)

235mm (9¼ ins)

Side View

310mm (12¼ ins)

Plan View

This cross piece may require the insertion of a matching length of wood dowelling as a reinforcement to prevent sagging.

Bedclothes Support.

All component parts are standard ¾ inch i.d. (19 mm. i.d.) polypropylene overflow water pipe system, with push-fit joints needing no glue.

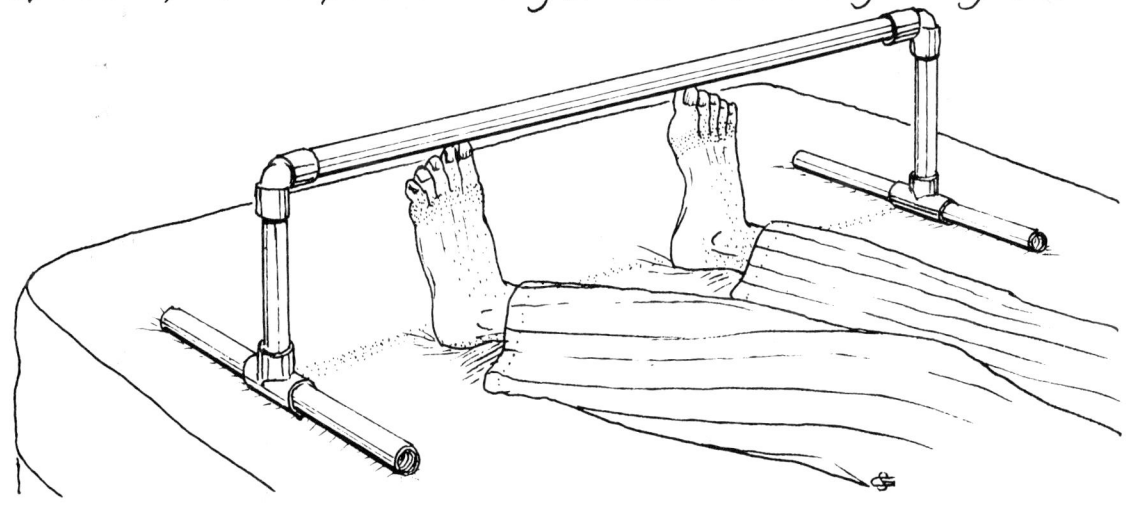

THE HOLDFAST

When using both hands, those who are able to do so may note that one hand, the left in the majority of us, is often holding an object static and steady, while the other hand is working on the object in some way, probably with a tool of some kind. It follows from this that a major problem for those who have full use of only one hand is the difficulty of holding on to an object whilst working on it with the 'good' hand. A vice or cramp may be able to help solve this problem in some degree, but placing an object in a vice or cramp with one hand only is no easy task in itself, although it may be eased by the judicious use of one of the re-useable adhesive putties, such as Blu-Tack, or a double-sided self-adhesive tape. Furthermore a vice or cramp can be disastrously hard on soft or delicate objects.

This design aims to provide a device which will hold most everyday objects steady, either horizontally or vertically, so that they can be worked on in some way. It acts by wrapping a length of two inch (25 mm) wide webbing around the object and then tensioning the webbing so that the object is held firmly, but relatively kindly, either horizontally against the Tensioner's side members, or vertically against two detachable pegs, between which the webbing passes and changes aspect from horizontal to vertical.

The Base of the Holdfast must be attached firmly to a stable work surface and probably the most convenient way of doing this is by means of one or more G-cramps. However, the Base may be screwed or bolted down if a permanent position can be provided.

The crucial component of the Holdfast is the Webbing Tensioner, which is a form of buckle and, indeed, could be used independently in other situations, through which the webbing can be drawn into tension and be held so until released by pressure on a conveniently placed bar.

The Webbing Tensioner has five component parts, two of which, the Side Supports, are identical and cut from 18 mm ($\frac{3}{4}$ inch) plywood. A slightly lesser thickness, if more convenient, would be adequate. There is only one moving part, which is the Outer Tube and this is made from a 70mm ($2\frac{3}{4}$ inches) length of 39 mm ($1\frac{1}{2}$ inch) internal diameter plastic water pipe, cut once longitudinally, so that its circumference can be opened to provide a snap fit over the Inner Tube. The Inner Tube is also a

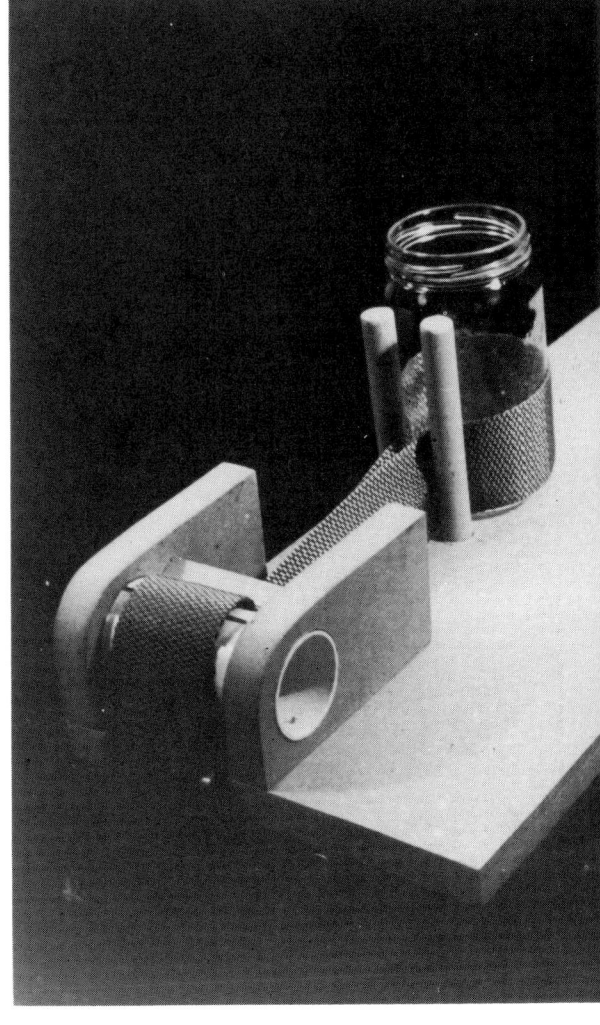

The Holdfast holding a jam jar vertically.

piece of the same size, 39 mm ($1\frac{1}{2}$ inch) internal diameter, plastic water pipe, but measuring 106 mm ($4\frac{3}{16}$ inches) in length. Two slots are cut in each of these two tubes, the slots being positioned in such a way that they do not quite coincide. When the webbing passing through them is brought into tension, the Outer Tube slides around the Inner and the webbing is jammed between the edges of an

THE HOLDFAST.

This shows the device in its vertical holding mode, a jar secured against the two detachable pegs.

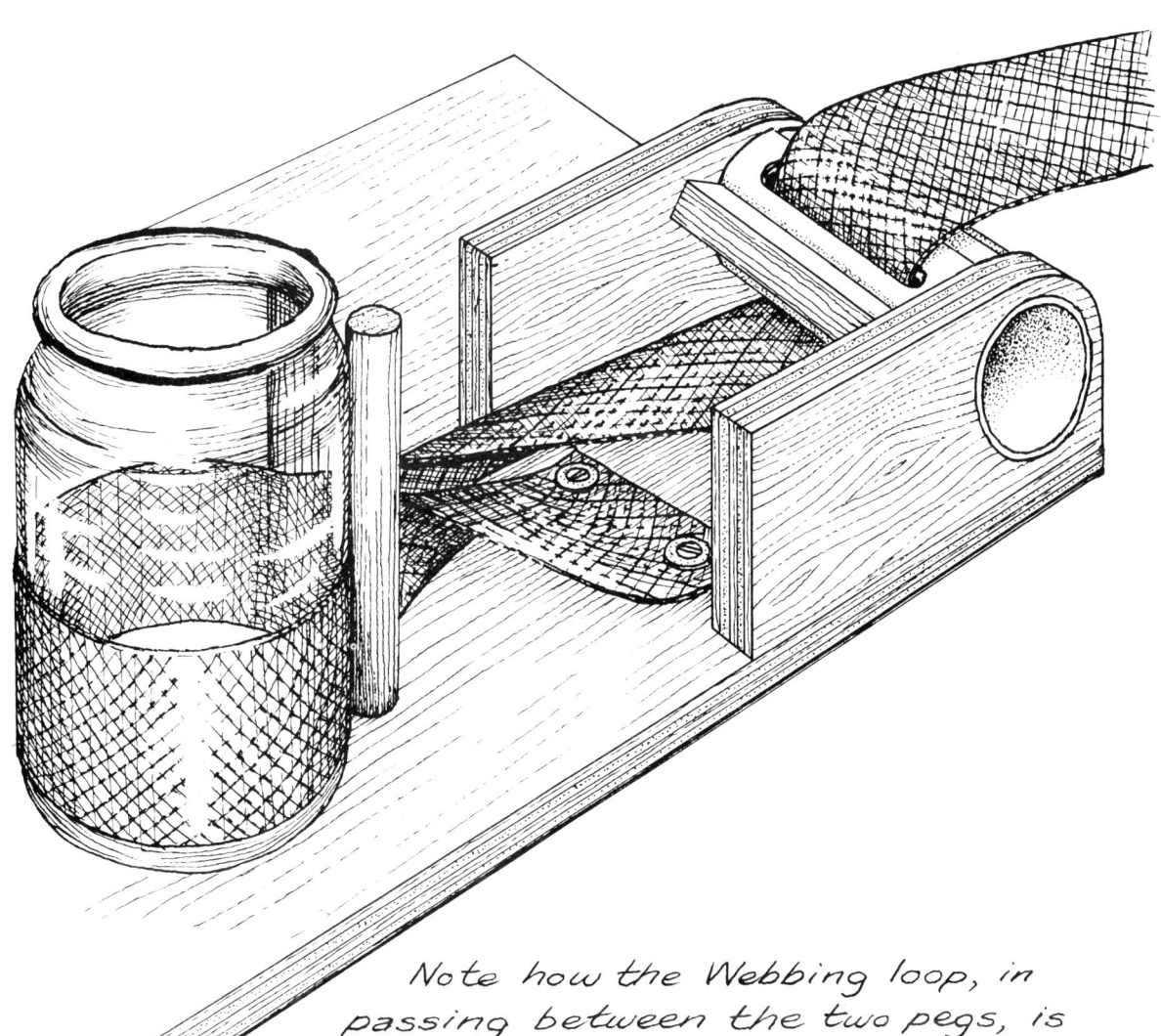

Note how the Webbing loop, in passing between the two pegs, is turned through a right angle, from horizontal to vertical.

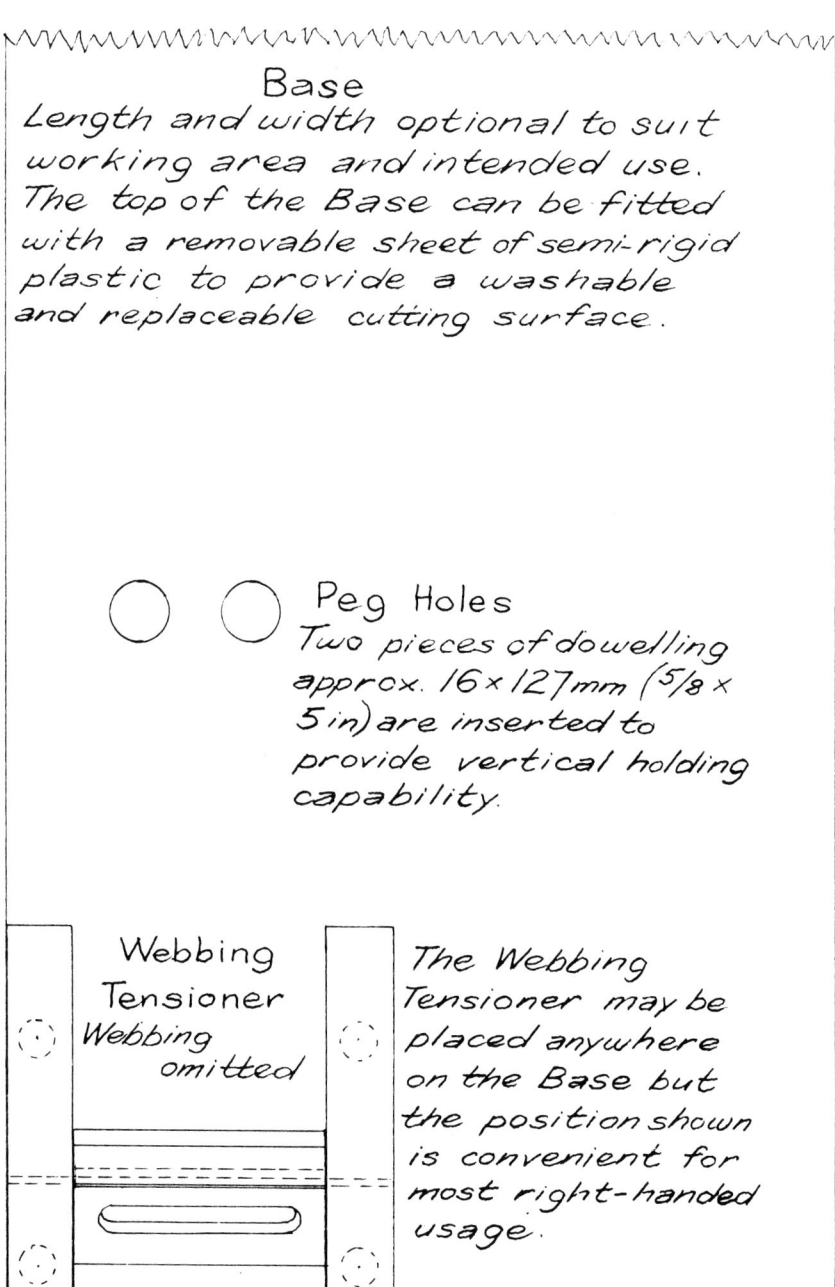

Base
Length and width optional to suit working area and intended use. The top of the Base can be fitted with a removable sheet of semi-rigid plastic to provide a washable and replaceable cutting surface.

Peg Holes
Two pieces of dowelling approx. 16 × 127mm (⅝ × 5 in) are inserted to provide vertical holding capability.

Webbing Tensioner
Webbing omitted

The Webbing Tensioner may be placed anywhere on the Base but the position shown is convenient for most right-handed usage.

THE HOLDFAST
General Arrangement ~ Plan ~ Scale ½

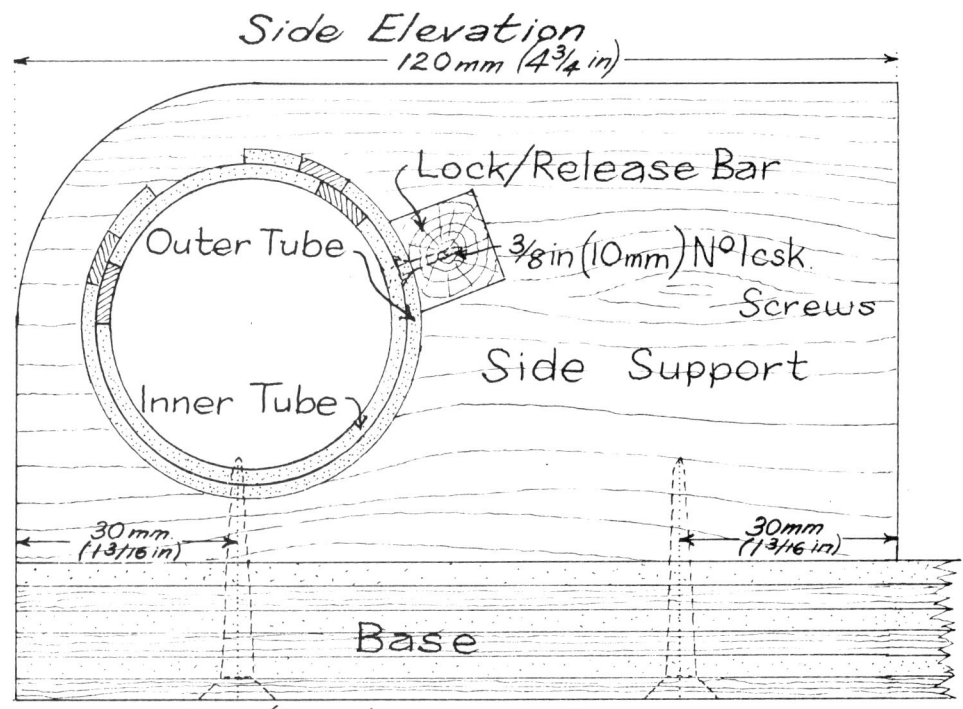

Side Elevation

120mm (4¾ in)

Lock/Release Bar

Outer Tube

⅜in (10mm) Nº1 csk. Screws

Side Support

Inner Tube

30 mm (1 3/16 in)

30mm (1 3/16 in)

Base

1¼ in (32mm) Nº8 csk. Screws

Note: the Outer Tube is a snap fit over the Inner Tube and is free to rotate between Side Supports.

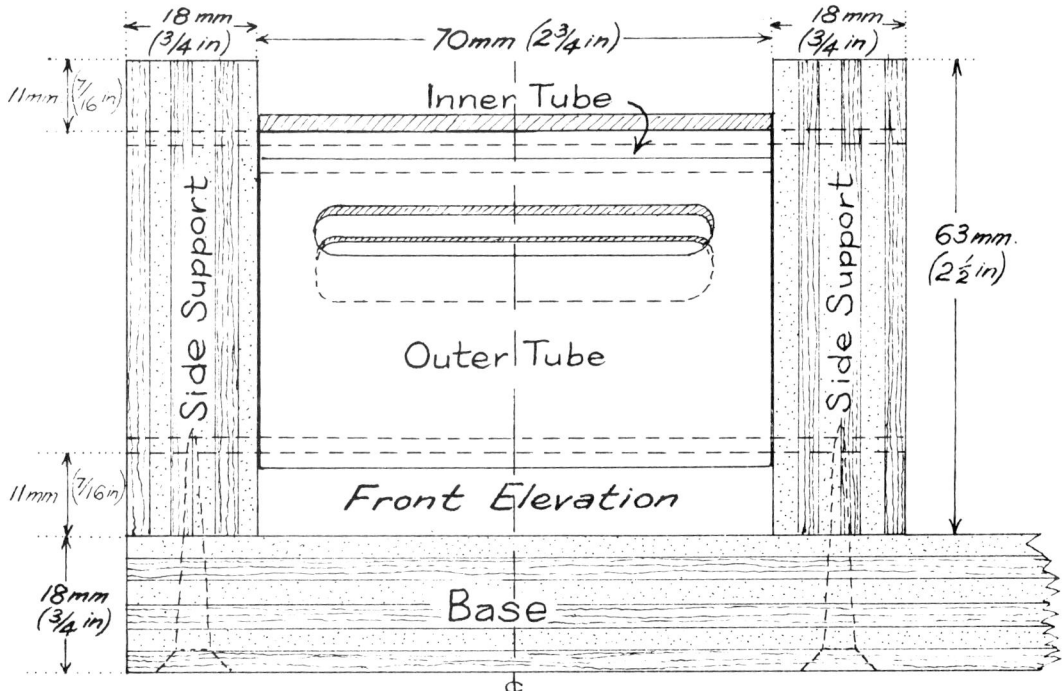

18 mm (¾ in)

70mm (2¾ in)

18 mm (¾ in)

11mm (7/16 in)

Inner Tube

63 mm (2½ in)

Side Support

Side Support

Outer Tube

11mm (7/16 in)

Front Elevation

18 mm (¾ in)

Base

Note: two of the Screws holding Base to Side Supports pass through Inner Tube to prevent it rotating.

Webbing Tensioner – General Arrangement.

Tensioner Components

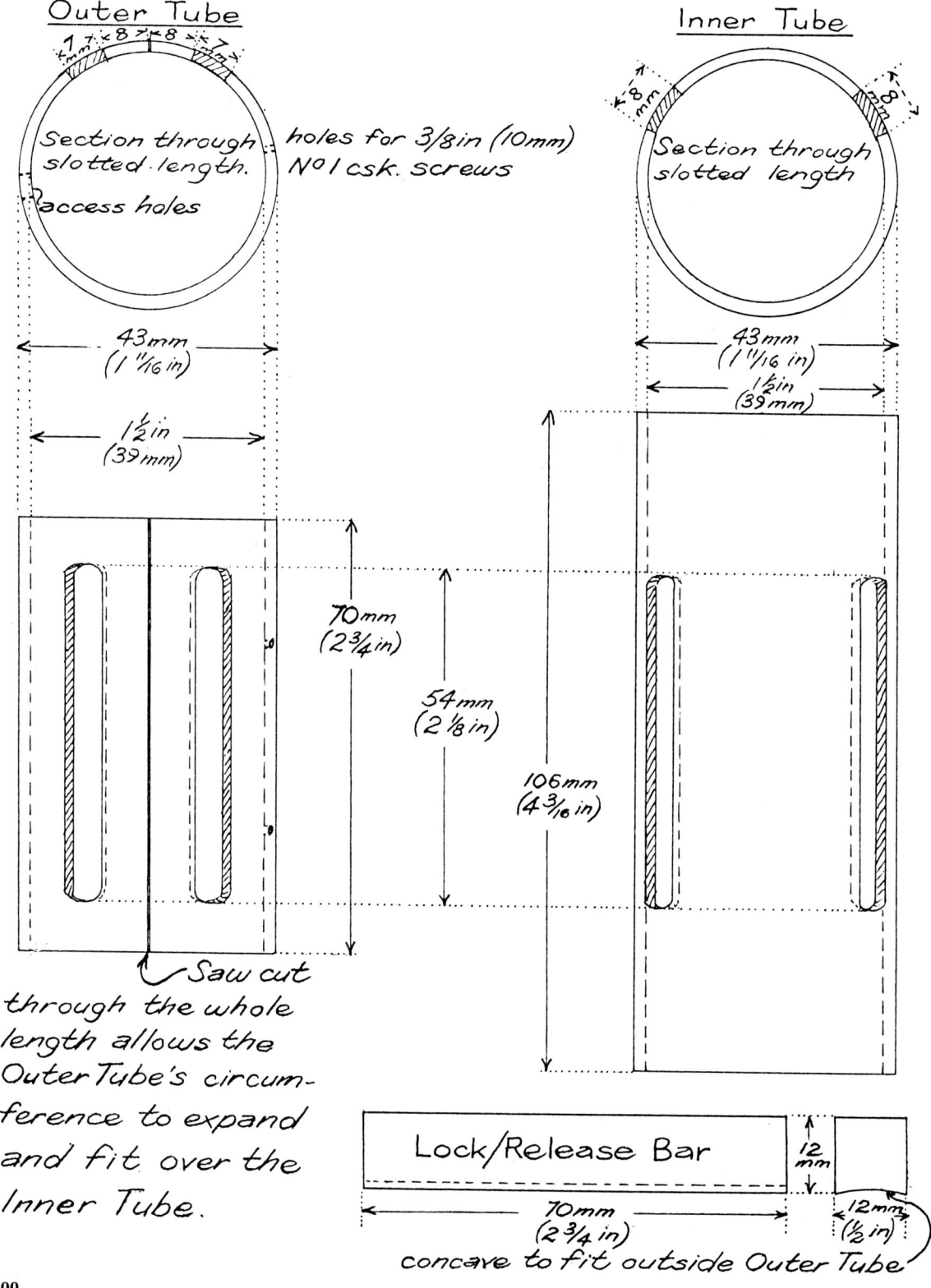

Outer Tube

Section through slotted length.

access holes

holes for 3/8in (10mm) Nº1 csk. screws

43mm (1 ¹¹/₁₆ in)

1½in (39mm)

70mm (2¾in)

Saw cut

through the whole
length allows the
Outer Tube's circum-
ference to expand
and fit over the
Inner Tube.

Inner Tube

Section through slotted length

43mm (1 ¹¹/₁₆ in)

1½in (39mm)

54mm (2⅛in)

106mm (4³/₁₆ in)

Lock/Release Bar

12mm

70mm (2¾in)

12mm (½in)

concave to fit outside Outer Tube

The Path of the Webbing through the Tensioner.

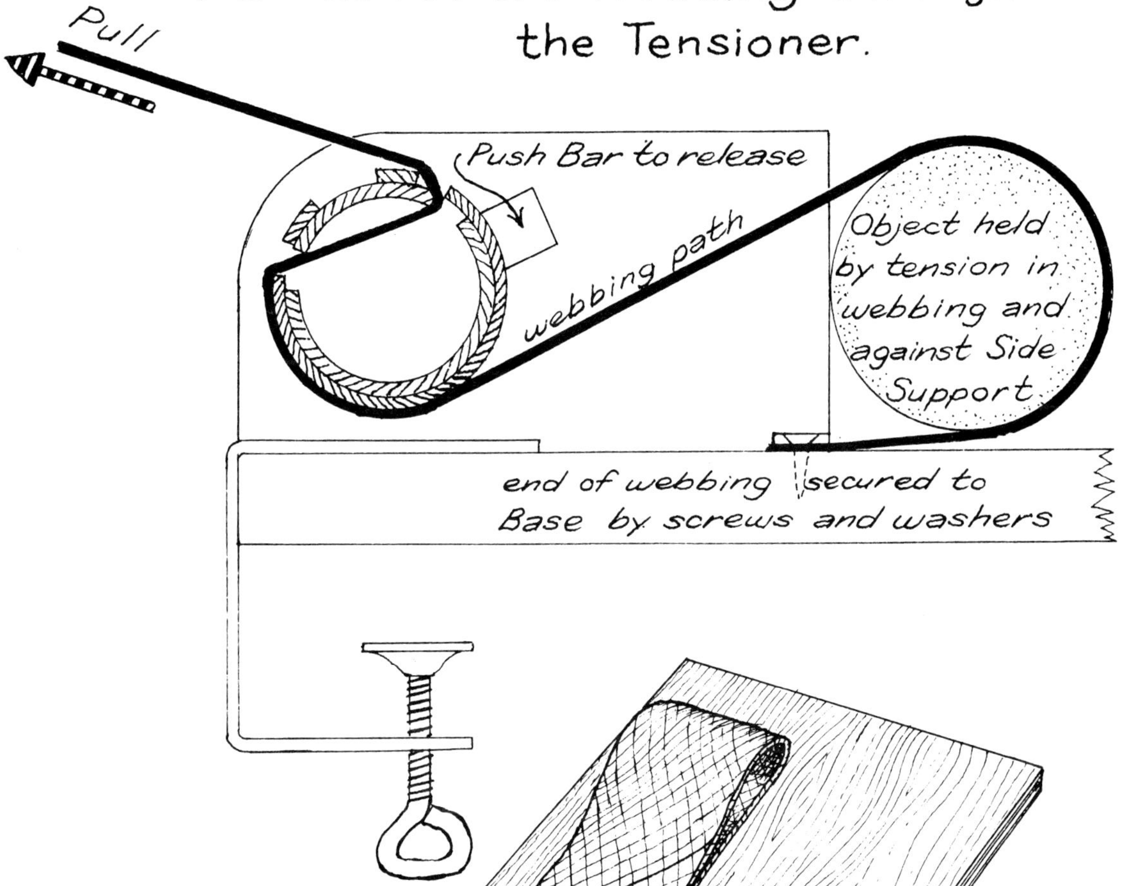

Pull

Push Bar to release

webbing path

Object held by tension in webbing and against Side Support

end of webbing secured to Base by screws and washers

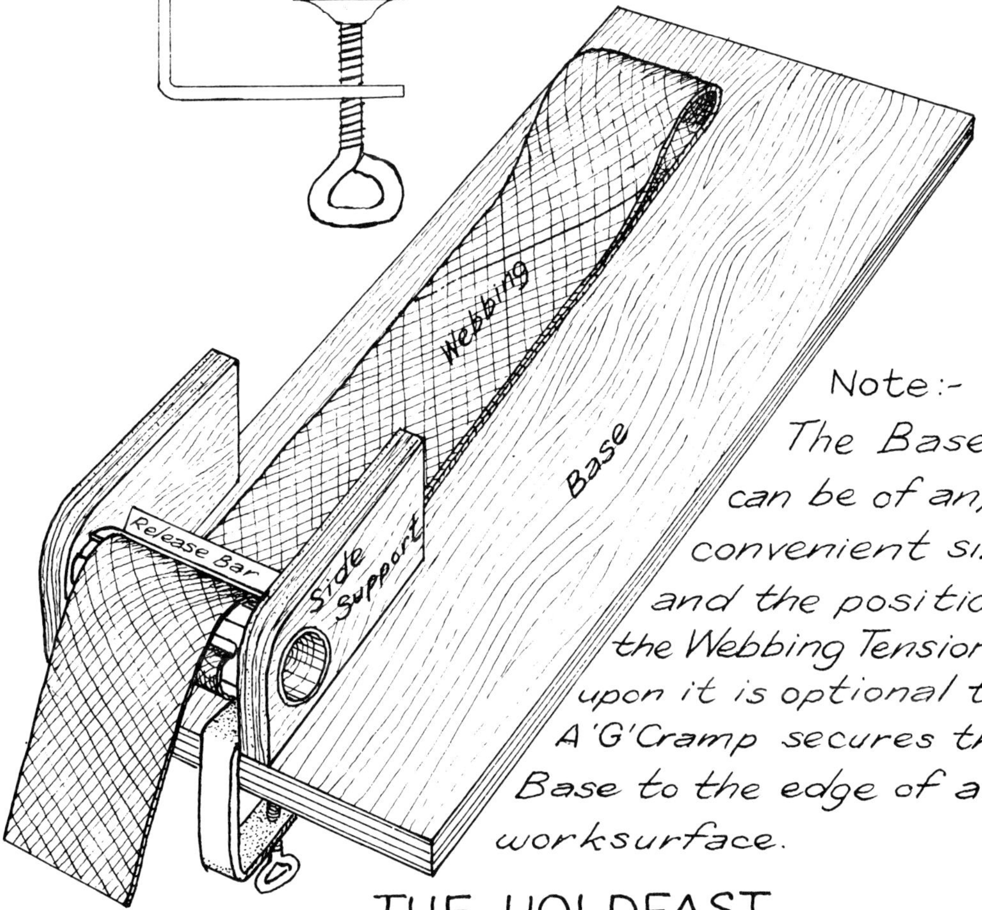

Webbing

Base

Release Bar

Side Support

Note:-
The Base can be of any convenient size and the position of the Webbing Tensioner upon it is optional too. A 'G' Cramp secures the Base to the edge of a worksurface.

THE HOLDFAST

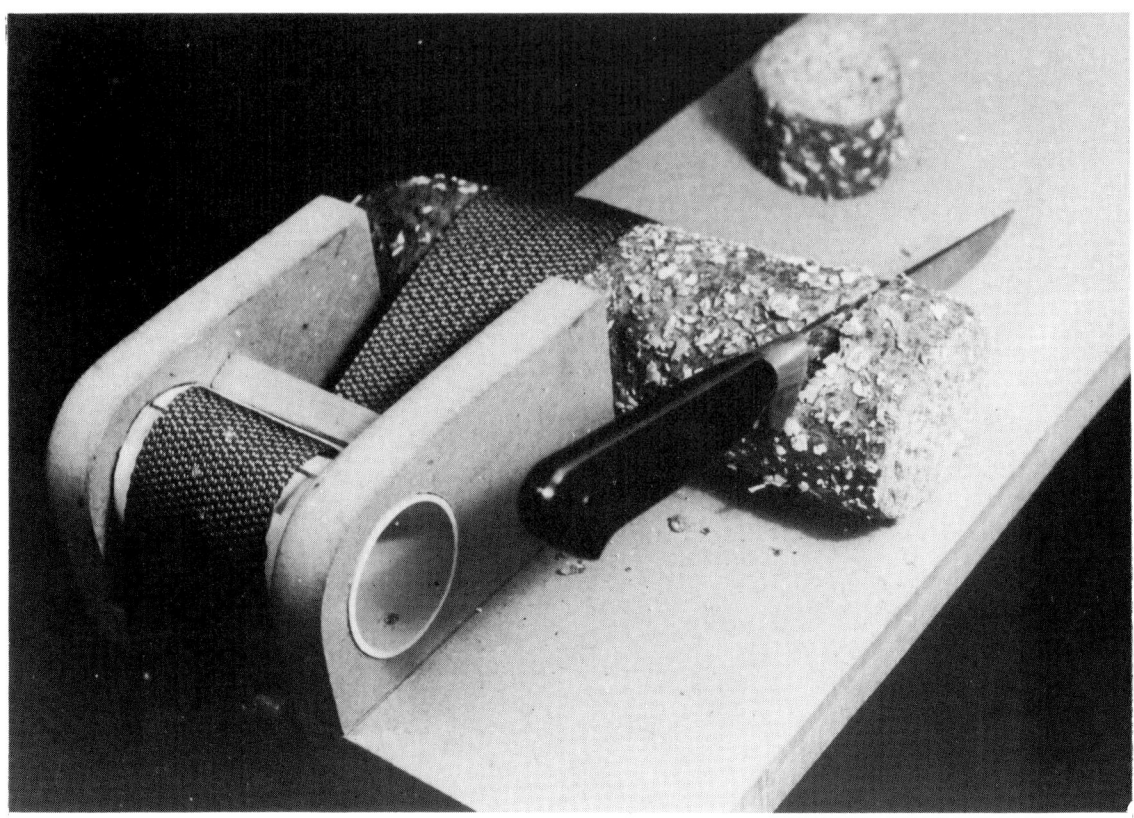

The Holdfast holding a French loaf for cutting.

inner and an outer slot. A Lock/Release Bar, made of 12 mm ($\frac{1}{2}$ inch) square section hardwood, is screwed to the upper part of the Outer Tube and provides the means of releasing the tension in the webbing by pushing the Bar downward. Similarly, the webbing can be locked at any point by pulling the Bar upward.

The upper surface of the Base can be protected by fitting to it a piece of plastic semi-rigid sheet, cut appropriately to size, which is easily washable and when cutting on it repeatedly has rendered a replacement necessary, this can be effected inexpensively.

The type of webbing used is of no great consequence, except that, if unusually thick, the Tensioner slots may have to be made wider. Webbing woven from man-made fibres will last better and is easily washable, but ex War Department cotton webbing is still available at very low cost, although it may need washing before it is used. Webbing 25 mm (2 inches) wide is well-suited for this purpose, and is widely available for use in car safety belts and upholstery. Other widths can be used, however, with appropriate adjustment of the Tensioner widths. In the kitchen the Holdfast will hold, say, a loaf, a salami sausage or a cucumber, firmly in a horizontal position so that slices can be cut. It will also hold a jar, tin, box or canister vertically upright against the two pegs set into appropriately placed holes in the Base, whilst contents are added or removed. Other uses in other situations, such as a workshop, can easily be imagined.

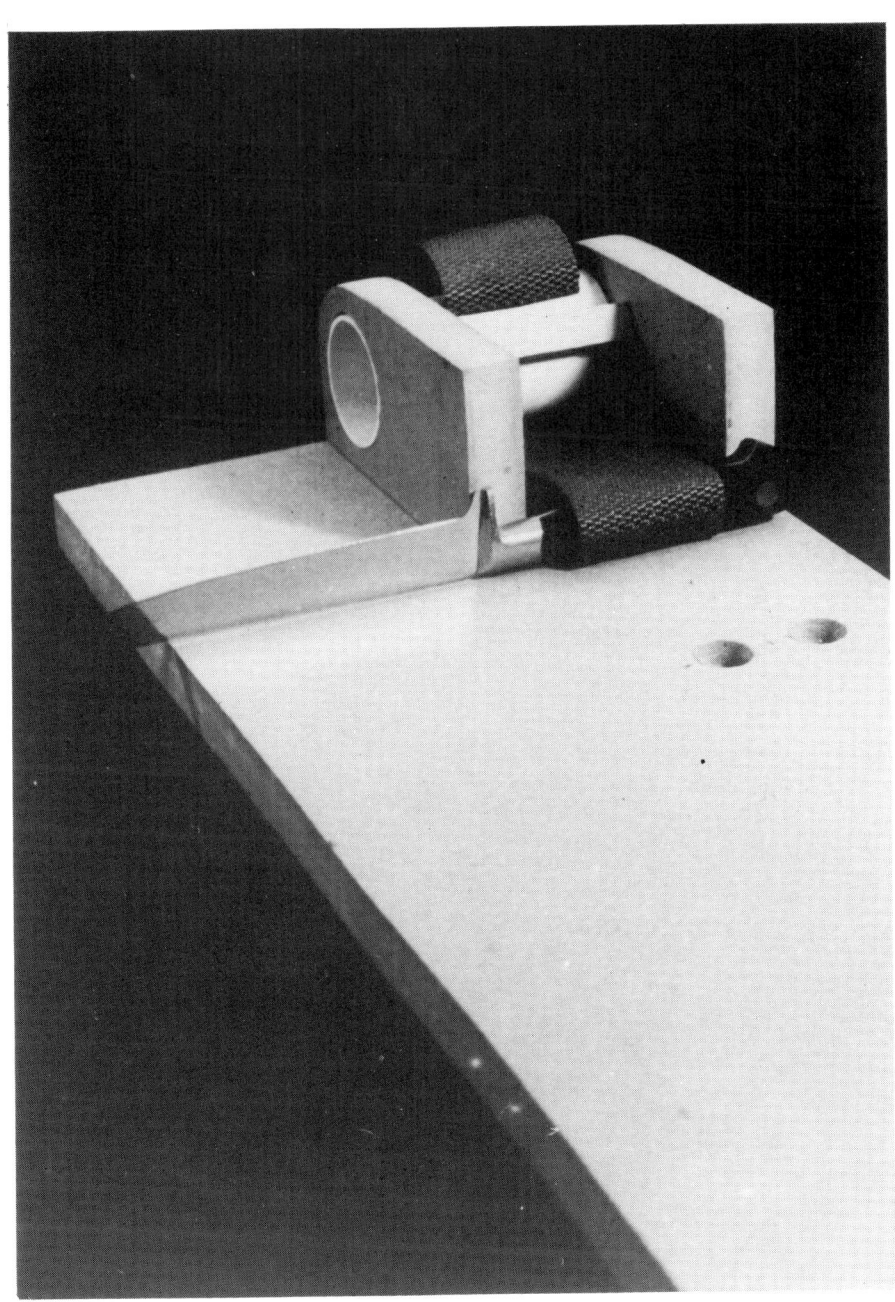

The Holdfast holding a knife horizontally, cutting
edge upward, ready for scraping vegetables.

ADVICE ON FINDING HELPFUL HANDYMEN

The emphasis throughout this book has been upon the making of the devices described, but it may well happen that a disabled person will find in the preceding pages an aid which could be helpful and feel frustrated by being unable to make it and knowing nobody who could do so. Here are a few suggestions for overcoming this problem by seeking practical help locally.

First consider carefully how difficult it seems to be to make the item you want. If it is quite simple, there is a good chance that someone with a different disability might be able to make it for you. In the UK the Department of Health and Social Services runs numerous Day Centres for the disabled, which are often provided with well-equipped workshops. Other countries have similar facilities under the auspices of different organizations, but they are all there to be helpful. A list of such organizations is included in the Appendix which follows.

Even the most difficult project in this book is well within the capability of the Craft Department of a senior school. Often the older pupils are delighted to have a really useful and practical project to pursue and, once they have made one successful device, they will be keen to have a try at making others. To make the first contact it is probably best to write briefly to the Head Teacher, explaining that you have a handicap and the means of at least partially overcoming it if someone capable of providing and using the necessary tools will help. In many cases no more than that will bring an eager youngster to your door.

Many Education Authorities, in the UK and elsewhere, run evening classes for adults, often in local schools, frequently including such crafts as woodwork, metalwork and upholstery. The supervisors of most such centres could find volunteers to make aids from among both pupils and instructors. Information about such classes and the names of appropriate contacts are often published in local newspapers, and a letter or a telephone call to a local newspaper or radio station seeking such help can often work wonders.

Other potential sources of help include your local church, Scout and Guide groups, Citizen's Advice Bureaux, Youth Clubs and many others. There are just two simple rules to remember in this situation:

1. Do not be too shy or too proud to ask for help – everyone needs a helping hand at some time and most people will respond eagerly if they know they will not be rebuffed.

2. Always offer to pay for at least the materials used. A willing helper should not have to pay for the privilege and will be more happy and able to help you or someone else again if expenses are met.

APPENDIX
Organizations which Offer Advice
and Support to the Disabled

Australia

Australian Red Cross Society,
200 Clarendon Street,
EAST MELBOURNE,
Victoria 3002.

National Committee of Independent Living Centres,
P.O. Box 351,
RYDE,
New South Wales 2112.

Independent Living Centre,
52 Thistlewaite Street,
SOUTH MELBOURNE,
Victoria 3205.

Independent Living Centre,
3 Lemnos Street,
Shenton Park,
PERTH,
Western Australia 6008.

Australian Council of Rehabilitation of Disabled
  (ACROD),
P.O. Box 60,
CURTIN,
ACT 2605.

Technical Aid to the Disabled,
P.O. Box 108,
RHYDE,
New South Wales 2112.

Disabled Persons Services,
  (Central Information Service),
'MAWARRA',
50/60 Albert Street,
BRISBANE,
Queensland 4000.

Queensland Disability Information and Resources
  Centre,
195 Giles Street,
ADELAIDE,
South Australia 5000.

Canada

The Canadian Red Cross Society,
1800 Alta Vista Drive,
OTTAWA,
Ontario K1G 4J5.

Disabled Living Resource Centre,
Kinsman Rehabilitation Foundation,
2256 West 12th Avenue,
VANCOUVER V6K 2N5.

Sunny Aids for Living Centre,
University of Toronto,
2075 Bayview Avenue,
TORONTO,
Ontario M4N 3M5.

Canadian Rehabilitation Council for the Disabled,
One Younge Street,
Suite 2110,
TORONTO,
Ontario M5E 1E5.

Technical Aids and Systems for the Handicapped
  Inc. (T.A.S.H.),
70 Gibson Drive,
MARKHAM,
Ontario L3R 462.

Republic of Ireland

Aids Information Service,
National Rehabilitation Board,
25 Clyde Road,
DUBLIN 4.

Disabled Aid (Ireland) Ltd.,
Aids and Equipment Centre (Commercial),
33 Charlemont Street,
DUBLIN 2.

New Zealand

The New Zealand Red Cross Society,
Red Cross House,
14 Hill Street,
WELLINGTON 1.

Disabled Living Centre/DPA N.Z. Inc.,
Tauranga Region,
Cnr 4th Avenue and Devonport Road,
P.O. Box 1135,
TAURANGA.

Independent Living Centre Inc.,
14 Erson Avenue,
P.O. Box 24/042 Royal Oak,
AUCKLAND 5.

Disabled Living Centre,
Aids Display and Information,
13 Milton Street,
P.O. Box 146,
HAMILTON.

Abilities Hawkes Bay Inc.,
208 Nelson Street South,
HASTINGS.

Aid Information Centre,
Rehabilitation League,
Leyland Street,
Onekawa,
P.O. Box 1043,
NAPIER.

Taranaki Disabled Living Centre,
28 Young Street,
P.O. Box 587,
NEW PLYMOUTH.

Kinross House Resource Centre Inc.,
Independent Living For the Disabled and the
   Elderly
P.O. Box 438,
BLENHEIM.

Independent Living Resource Centre,
Community Services,
Dunedin Hospital,
DUNEDIN.

Mosgiel Disabled Living Centre,
Taieri Physically Disabled Persons Group Inc.,
P.O. Box 372,
c/o 34 Argyle Street,
Mosgiel,
OTAGO.

Disabled Persons Assembly (N.Z.) Inc.,
P.O. Box 27 – 186,
67 Hanky Street,
WELLINGTON.

United Kingdom

Age Concern England,
Bernard Sunley House,
60 Pitcairn Road,
MITCHAM,
Surrey CR4 3LL.

Arthritis Care,
6 Grosvenor Crescent,
LONDON SW1X 7ER.

British Limbless Ex-Servicemen's Association,
Frankland Moore House,
185–187 High Road,
CHADWELL HEATH,
Essex.

British Red Cross Society,
9 Grosvenor Crescent,
LONDON SW1X 7EJ.

The Disabled Living Foundation,
380–384 Harrow Road,
LONDON W9 2HU.

Help the Aged,
St James' Walk,
LONDON EC1R 0BE.

National Association of Citizen's Advice Bureaux,
Middleton House,
115–123 Pentonville Road,
King's Cross,
LONDON N1 9LZ.

Physically Handicapped and Able-Bodied, (PHAB),
Tavistock House North,
Tavistock Square,
LONDON WC1 9HX.

Queen Elizabeth's Foundation for the Disabled,
LEATHERHEAD,
Surrey KT22 0BN.

Royal Association for Disability and Rehabilitation
   (RADAR),
25 Mortimer Street,
LONDON W1N 8AB.

Women's Royal Voluntary Service Trust,
17 Old Park Lane,
LONDON W1Y 4AJ.

NOTE:
Probably the most readily available source of help
and advice for handicapped people in the UK is the
local Council's Social Services Department, which
normally appears in the telephone directory under
the name of the County Council.

United States of America

American Red Cross,
17th and D Streets, N.W.,
WASHINGTON,
D.C. 2006.

Pam Assistance Centre,
601 West Maple Street,
LANSING,
Michigan 48906.

HYGEIA (Commercial Centre),
The Accessibility House,
582 Westbury Avenue,
Carle Place,
NEW YORK,
NY 71514.

Rehabilitation International,
25 East 21st Street,
NEW YORK,
NY 10010.

Index

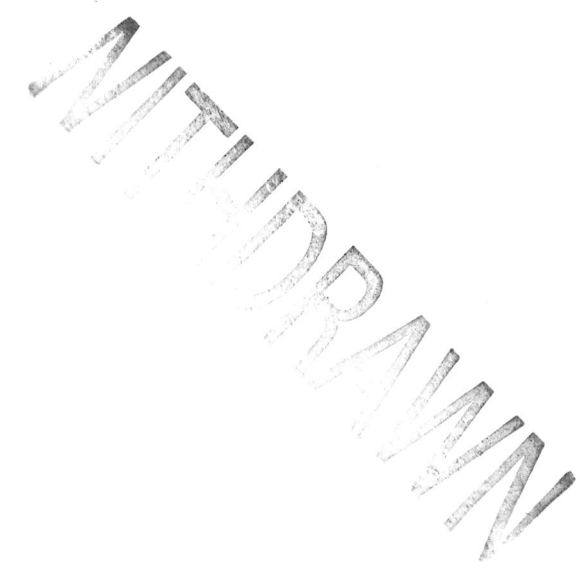